THE TAO

How to achieve health and long life using the Taoist dietary system of Ch'ang Ming.

THE TAO OF LONG LIFE

The Chinese Art of Ch'ang Ming

by

CHEE SOO

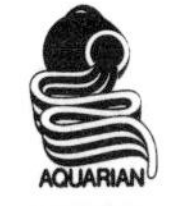

THE AQUARIAN PRESS
Wellingborough, Northamptonshire

First published 1979
First Trade Paperback Edition 1982

© CHEE SOO 1979

This book is sold subject to the condition that it shall not, by way of trade or otherwise, be lent, re-sold, hired out, or otherwise circulated without the publisher's prior consent in any form of binding or cover other than that in which it is published and without a similar condition including this condition being imposed on the subsequent purchaser.

British Library Cataloguing in Publication Data

Soo, Chee
The Tao of long life.
1. Diet 2. Food, Natural
3. Philosophy, Taoist
I. Title
613.2'6 RA784

ISBN 0-85030-320-6

Printed and bound in Great Britain.

Contents

To all Humanity

Those who are fit are not necessarily healthy
Those that are good are not necessarily virtuous
Both need to change their attitudes to life.

Let Ch'ang Ming safeguard your body
You concentrate on controlling your own mind
The Tao will constantly look after your spirit.

Chee Soo

Foreword

You say to yourself, "What a lovely Christmas it is going to be", then two days before the event you go down with 'flu.

It happens

As regularly as clockwork a migraine attack comes on each weekend, and so you find it impossible to plan your holidays in advance.

It happens

You get the offer of a lovely cottage in the country, but dare not take advantage of it for you suffer from severe hay fever all through the summer.

It happens

The sufferers from arthritis, rheumatism and cancer all dread the coming of November for it signifies the onset of intense aches and pains, sleepless nights, and a complete lack of energy.

It happens

Yes! It happens to millions and millions of people all over the world, not just occasionally, but every single day of the year, and there are many sick and suffering all around you even as you read this. Almost every house in any town has someone suffering from something or another, even if it is only a few spots, a boil, stomach upset, a cold or a mild headache. On any day, look at the people walking along the streets, notice how many appear pale, grim and forlorn, as though life held no meaning and no hope and they were expecting the end of their life to come at any minute. What a way to live, what a way to survive; surely being born holds a greater meaning than this?

Haven't you ever asked yourself why the people in the West are so unhealthy? Do you take your illnesses for granted? Do you *expect* to be ill occasionally, to get colds and 'flu every winter? Do you take it for granted that when the winter comes some of the old folk will die from hypothermia? Do you expect your child to have tonsilitis, bad teeth, diarrhoea at some time? Do you really expect all this, even though we are supposed to be living in a scientific world where the top technicians and doctors are SUPPOSED to know all the answers and have a great understanding of the universe?

If you really expect all this, than you have completely the wrong attitude to life, and either do not know or have forgotten the true way of life and the real reason why you were born, and are lacking faith in the works of the Supreme Spirit (Yuhuang Tati) or God. We human beings were never meant to suffer ill health at all and no one should ever *expect* to be sick, during their life on earth, for if the delicate mechanism of the human body is looked after properly and correctly nourished with the right foods, it can continually adjust itself so that the balance is maintained internally in accordance with the essential principles of the Yin and Yang, and so enjoy permanent good health.

If, however, you eat the rubbish that commonly passes for food in the West, and refuse to change your ideas then you can fully expect bad health, sickness, aches, pains, and drugs to be a part of your daily life until you reach the end of your days here on earth. If you are happy with your present circumstances and way of life, and are quite ready to face the dreary prospect of ill health in the days to come, then do not read any more of this book, for it is not meant for you. We do, however, sincerely wish you the best of luck in the future, and hope that your suffering, no matter how small, will at least be of short duration.

On the other hand, if you hate the thought of being sick and of having to take drugs for the rest of your life, and are ready and willing to take practical steps to ensure a happy, healthy future for yourself, then read on, and join our family of millions. If you persevere, then your own improved health will be an encouragement to pass on the word to your relatives and neighbours and other people that you may meet along the pathway of your life, so that they too may enjoy a happier and healthier existence.

Basically there are three kinds of sickness that can affect the human body and they come under these categories, physical sickness, mental illness, and spiritual deterioration. These are so closely interrelated so that it is possible to heal any one of these, but in the process, all can be cured simultaneously. In this modern world we only have to look at the statistics, to realise that with continually increasing laws and regulations and mounting pressures, ill health is on the upsurge and violence is becoming more and more widespread. Most people are appalled at these symptoms of decline, yet do not bother to seek the true cause of them.

This is apparent when you consider that not so long ago cancer was almost unheard of, yet today one in every three persons in Britain and the United States of America has this illness in one form or another. Still the Western world has discovered no cure for it, and does not properly understand what causes it, although certain things are known to spark if off or aggravate it. In China, by contrast, it is recognised that due to a lack of internal energy (Nei Pu Chi) and external or macrocosmic energy (Ching Sheng Li) within the tissues and nervous systems of the body induces a state of internal hypothermia, which so weakens the body that it is unable to fight off the growth of the cancer. Correct this equilibrium and the cancer dies, or better still correct the eating habits and cancer will not develop. In other words, remove the cause of the weakness and the ill effects and symptoms will not appear.

In a report published by the National Health Federation of California in 1975 it was stated that it had been found that artificially fluoridated water encourages cancer. Fluoride and chloride numb the tissues and nervous systems of the human body and thereby produce ideal conditions for a cancer growth to flourish. The number of deaths from cancer was well above the national average for the U.S.A. in cities such as Chicago, Philadelphia and Baltimore, that had fluoridated their water, but was equal or below the average in, for instance, Los Angeles, San Antonio and San Diego which had not introduced fluoridation. Various other contaminants that are added to or that find their way into drinking water, such as chlorine, chlorinated hydrocarbons and pesticides, were also found to be linked to cancer. So there is a lesson to be learnt from this, always ensure that you boil your drinking water.

The well-known pesticide, DDT, which has been used to increase crop yields, has been found to cause infertility in human beings, it also increased the toxic content to a level higher than the tolerances permitted by the World Health Organisation for milk products. In a mother it may increase the toxic residue of her own milk to more than sixteen times that of cows milk, and could therefore endanger the health of her own child. These are just a couple of examples of the harm that chemicals can do.

The colourings, flavourings, additives, preservatives, artificial fruit acids and so on that are contained in the packaged and canned foods on sale in supermarkets and shops greatly add to the amount of chemicals regularly consumed, plus the drugs taken for illnesses, by the average Westerner. Added to all this, a great many things that are eaten contain residues of pesticides, detergents, and so forth. The strain of the human body trying to cope with such toxic matter that you consume every day of your life is considerable and in addition, there are the natural toxins and acids that the body produces during its own daily work which weaken the metabolism and make it a prey to ill health when it need not be.

We who follow the ancient Chinese Arts are very wary about the amount of dairy products we give to babies and children, for we have an old saying, "If you want your child to grow up looking and acting like an animal, then feed it cow's milk or goat's milk from the day it is born". In China it is a well-known fact that cow's milk dulls the mind, and goat's milk makes a child stubborn, so, in order that children should have the best nourishment right from the start, even before it is born, the mother should herself follow a natural healthy diet, and Ch'ang Ming is the answer. As for taking drugs during pregnancy, the thalidomide tragedy is or should be sufficient warning against that.

Don't listen to the scientists; ignore the constant flow of words from the politicians; and endeavour to live your life according to the laws of the Supreme Spirit, who controls all things in the universe, and learn to follow the true way (Tao) of your natural life here on earth.

Though men may disagree, women are spiritually, mentally and physically stronger than they are. Women also live longer than men—on an average about five years longer, and they are the backbone of every nation, for they run the home, make sure all the bills are paid, and govern and control the growth and the health of the children. Most important of all, it is they who do the shopping, decide what to buy and plan the meals of the family. Woman is the kingpin of her own health, her husband and her family, and, if anyone can persuade them to eat and drink the right things, she can. What a terrific responsibility she has, for the future health of herself, her husband and her children, and thus of future generations, is truly in her hands, and what she purchases for her shopping basket. Though this is not to deny that men also follow the Tao, and perhaps have been able to persuade their wives to do likewise, and this is true harmony between opposites as it should always be, and let it be yours as well for this is the true order of the universe.

This morning I had a telephone call from a woman who has suffered with very bad nerves for over ten years, and it has got so bad that her sons and daughters have all left home, and her husband has moved into another bedroom and no longer speaks to her. She has been off her food for a long time, and she asked for help, in response to which I explained to her the need for changing her diet and using some herbs. She replied, "What good is eating the Ch'ang Ming way, i.e., according to the Chinese Health Arts, to me for I need help, not a diet" and she could not see that eating properly and sensibly was no more difficult, though far more beneficial, than the drugs she has been taking over the years, and which are doing her no good at all.

Food is extremely important and fundamental to human survival, and we cannot exist without it, either physically, mentally or spiritually (for the spirit absorbs energy through the soul from the body as well as from heaven). Food supplies the nutrition that supports the lifelines of the human body, and through it we either gain or lose energy, depending on the particular food that is eaten. This energy, and the quality and quantity of it, are so vital that if you lack energy, you can have a nervous breakdown, while, if you have the right balance you will attain not only dynamic concentration and control but constant good health.

Therefore if you adopt correct eating and drinking habits not only will you completely change your life, and feel much better within yourself, but your family and friends will notice the alertness and sparkle in your eyes, and the beautiful and healthy texture of your skin. You will find that your mind will become more relaxed, that you will change your ways of thinking, and that you will sleep more soundly and deeper. Spiritually too, you will gain greater strength, and as your whole outlook on life changes, you will find that you are increasingly prepared to help and serve others, and will get great joy and happiness in doing so.

A few hundred years ago, natural grain foods, fruit and vegetables, untampered with by man, were the normal food of the day with the addition of many herbs that were used to give an extra flavour to the meals. Though only the rich could afford the dearer meat products in those days, this was not entirely to the disadvantage of the poor, for it meant that they kept to a more natural, and thus healthier diet, provided that they had enough to eat. Therefore they conformed to the natural order of life and the universal laws of the cosmos, and illnesses such as cancer were scarcely known.

Today few people follow the natural way of eating and drinking, and abide by the universal laws of nature, for they have been enticed, coaxed and coerced into eating all the wrong things by people whose only concern is to make more and more money, by playing upon the five senses. Food is made to look more attractive, by decoration and colouring, just to attract attention, some foods are prepared in such a way that their aroma will torment your sense of smell. In the hot weather you will be attracted to the ice-cream van because you feel you need something cool and refreshing. So all your senses are played havoc with, for the sake of selling more and more.

Eating at regular times each day, whether you feel hungry or not, is a bad habit that has to be conquered. This may not be easy, for you may have meals prepared for you, either at home or elsewhere, and considerations of courtesy may make it difficult to leave or refuse what you do not have the appetite for or do not really like.

Some people seek to model their diet according to various "scientific principles" which is to say, on fat or calorie content, or according to some new fad. A few years ago, for instance, there was a fad in the U.S.A. for eating nothing but brown rice. None of these quirks of the principles of nature have any value, neither do they benefit the health of the human body, and they certainly have no practical foundation within nature, for they are one-sided and therefore out of balance. After all, it is the health of the individual that really matters, and that is the objective of Ch'ang Ming, which has been truly proven over thousands of years.

Then there are those we could call the "excusers", because they will always find an excuse not to eat the right things, even if it means that their health will improve. The most common excuse is that it costs too much to eat properly, when in fact eating the Ch'ang Ming way is much cheaper than following other inadequate dietary programmes. Some will tell you that they cannot stomach vegetables many of which they have doubtless never tried, and that they give them wind. Some will say that they would not dream of giving up fried food, when in fact it is only deep-fried food that needs to be wholly avoided: sauté or stir-fried foods are an acceptable part of a balanced diet.

Another excuse is that grain food is fattening and so they immediately come to the conclusion that they will lose their slim figures. The truth is that if you settle down to the Ch'ang Ming health diet you invariably lose weight for you will get rid of the toxins and acidity in the body, and you will come down to your natural body weight.

Many more excuses could be added to those mentioned here. It is amazing what lengths some people will go to to avoid trying something that will do them good, but in which they happen not to be interested at the time. It is easy when one is young and in a reasonable state of health, to act this way; but when the years have passed and the body begins to be racked with pain, and various other symptoms of illness begin to show, then, when it is almost too late, people begin desperately searching for a miracle cure.

There are, of course, those people who do not seek excuses, but simply shut their ears and close their eyes. They take the attitude that anything that seems newfangled to them, even though it may be a thousand years old, is not worth considering, or they may feel so depressed that they can think of nothing but of trying to "end it all"—not realising that in their next reincarnation after committing suicide, they would have to go through the same situation and circumstances again, to have the courage to finish what had begun; for all must follow their true destiny to the end, and they must learn that you cannot take life, not even their own, for only the Supreme Spirit has that right.

Then there are those who will never put themselves out at all for anyone or for anything, and are quite content to sit back and let everyone else do it all for them. They will bear the pain, play on it at times to get their own way, as long as they are waited on hand and foot, day in and day out. They are never happier than when everyone is chasing around for them, and taking care of their every need.

Then there is a small minority of people who close their minds, so that nothing will ever get through, and they will not do anything for anyone, will not accept anything at all not even advice, and so they become human skeletons, a bane to everyone around them, and slowly they lose all their friends, and sometimes their own kith and kin. Slowly they lose touch with the world around them and they no longer care or understand what is happening.

You may well recognise from your own personal experience the type of people described above. What is certain is that there are very many of them, and due to their attitude they do not live their life to the full. Large numbers of them can be said to do little more than exist, they give nothing and get very little out of life and so they restrict their own spiritual growth. Their attitudes may be the cause of misery, harassment, unhappiness and even ill health in others particularly those who should be closest to them. This is illustrated by the following cases.

Multiple Sclerosis

A husband brought his twenty-three year old wife along in a wheelchair to discuss whether the Chinese health arts could be of benefit to her. She had been incapacitated for over a year, having lost the use of her legs; but on hearing that she would be expected to change her eating and drinking habits, and on being given an outline of what this would mean, she flatly refused to change, even though her husband was quite willing to change his diet as well, so that they could both do it together. That was four years ago, and, as dedicated as he was, he eventually got fed up with lifting her in and out of bed and her wheelchair, taking her to the toilet, wheeling her everywhere and never going out himself. Eventually his own health broke down, and now he has left her.

In another case the husband had multiple sclerosis, and was slowly getting worse; he could hardly walk and then with extreme difficulty. He and his wife together decided that he should start the Ch'ang Ming health diet and Chinese herbal therapy (Ts'aoyao), but the wife refused to do the same. After a month she said that she could not cook one type of meal for herself and a different one for him, and she remained absolutely adamant that she would not change her own diet under any circumstances. So not only has she now penalised him for the rest of his life, but in addition she will have to nurse him continuously. In the not too distant future, he will have to give up his work, for his hands are slowly being affected. It is a great shame, for he was an excellent worker and organiser, and a first-class design engineer.

Epilepsy

A man used to have attacks of epilepsy at least once a month, but after sticking to his Ch'ang Ming diet he went nine months without having a single attack. However, one evening at a wedding celebration he was pressed into taking a small drink of alcohol to toast the bride and groom. When, shortly afterwards, he was crossing the road to his car, which was parked in a dimly lit suburban estate, he developed a bad attack, and in the semi-darkness a car hit him. He died, and all because of one little tot of alcohol.

Rheumatoid Arthritis

Two sisters, who lived together in Southern London, both suffered from rheumatoid arthritis, and both willingly started on the Ch'ang Ming health diet and Chinese herbal therapy. After about five years both were cured, but, whereas one sister never had time off from work, even though at times she suffered excruciating pain, the other sister always found an excuse not to go to work. Even though both are cured, the one sister is still constantly complaining of pains, and in over two years has not done a single day's work. So the other has to continue to support her. Perhaps one day the truth will come out; but the working sister is such a wonderful person that we are sure she will readily forgive. Maybe she already knows or has guessed, though she has never given her thoughts away in this respect. One day they will both have their Yin Kuo (retribution), when all the facts of their lives have been added up.

Heart Trouble

He had always been the life and soul of the party, and everyone was very surprised when one day he had a heart attack. His wife talked him into visiting a Ch'ang Ming consultant, which he did, aided by his wife's dedication, he religiously did as he had been instructed—except in one respect: he absolutely refused to give up his drink each evening with his circle of friends. The result was that he had a second stroke, is paralysed down one side of his body, and has extreme difficulty in walking without the use of his sticks. Needless to say, he is no longer the life and soul of the party, as he very rarely goes out; for without his sticks or his wife's support he cannot get about. Still, however, he has a tot of drink every night—but at home.

Ignorance, short-sightedness, ingratitude, dogmatism and foolishness—these are qualities that, as these cases illustrate, are all too prevalent. Trying to help others may sometimes seem a thankless task, bringing little reward; but do not be dismayed or discouraged, persevere, and, though not all will respond, some will. We should all seek to use our influence for good, in so far as we are able.

This foreword is unusual, and has been intentionally blunt, in the hope that the truth has made a deep impression, and pointed out the choice that faces each one of us: to continue following the lazy Western eating and drinking habits, which have a tendency to encourage illness and prevent one from fully realising one's mental and spiritual potential; or to eat and drink the Ch'ang Ming way and so come to enjoy continual good health and be able to fulfil one's inner self and to help and serve others. Yes! this is no ordinary book.

The Door is now open, the Way lies before you, and you are welcome to enter and join the millions who already share the universe with kind thoughts, good deeds, and enjoy a proper understanding of the underlying principles of nature, and so live close to heaven while still on earth.

Remember that we are all part of the Tao, and that our life, its structure, and our destiny was laid down long before we were born, even who our parents would be, what part of the world we would be born in, and the environment that would surround us. If we learn to accept all this, and work to the best of our ability, thinking and doing good whenever we can, then life will expand and new horizons open up for us so that we see all things that make up the universe: such as the ever present spiritual, mental and physical wonders that exist constantly in our daily life but to which most people are blind through living a life that is wrapped up in all the mundane concerns of a commercial world.

If your physical and mental activities take precedence over the spiritual side of your life then you will suffer physical hardships and mental anguish. In other words, you will create your own illness, for which the blame is entirely upon your own shoulders; but even at a very late stage it can be conquered, proving that by throwing open the mind, learning to live to the rules of the universe, and getting closer to the Supreme Spirit, all things are possible, and that miracles happen not only in the Bible and other holy books, but also in everyday life, if only you have the eyes to see and appreciate what is going on around you.

Those seeking a cure for any of their serious illnesses should first of all start to say their prayers regularly, and so become part of the spiritual life on earth; then, by changing their diet to the Ch'ang Ming principles and their outlook on life, their Yin world starts altering to a Yang one, and a new lease of life begins.

This is one of the many wonders of the Tao, of which we are all an integral part—come, start to recognise it.

Introduction

The average person eats simply to "fill a hole" and stay alive, and does not appreciate that the health of humanity depends on the goodness of the food consumed, and that any diet should be correctly balanced at all times. What is "correct" is naturally different for the individuals of each nation, their locality in the world, and where their ancestors came from. Through good, natural and wholesome food it is possible to obtain the correct balance of Yin and Yang, internally and externally, and to guard against and rectify any weaknesses that may have developed over the years.

Ch'ang Ming was developed by the Taoists between 10,000–5,000 BC, on the basis of the guidelines and foundations handed down to them by the "Sons of Reflected Light", a sect of people reputed to have been over seven feet in height, and who wore a type of clothing that had never before been seen in China. Where they came from is still a mystery, and perhaps we may never know the answer to this riddle, but on arrival in China they began to choose artisans and craftsmen from every known profession, selecting those of the highest intelligence. Having collected this band of people together, they began to instruct them in many different arts and crafts far in advance of anything else that existed in those far-off days. Many of them are still a long way ahead of anything that is in existence even to this present age.

To learn these arts and crafts thoroughly took many years, and many died without being able to completely master them. Even so, the knowledge was faithfully passed on to generation after generation, and so the work and the studies continued. Among the skills passed on were silk-weaving, pottery, glass and gunpowder making, and metal working; but most important of all was the enormous range of the health arts.

Down through the ages, great efforts have been made to carry on the good work; but, in the many years that have elapsed since the "Sons of Reflected Light" first came to China, some of their teachings may, even so, have been lost. Just how much, it is impossible to say, for there are no known written records from those early days.

The health arts that the "Sons of Reflected Light" brought to China eventually came to be known as the "Eight Strands of the Brocade" (Pa Chin Hsien), and even to this day, after thousands of years have passed, they are still known to the Chinese by that name. In the West these same arts are being used for the benefit of all who wish to avail themselves of them, and in London there is a health clinic where they are used to help, free of charge, sufferers of all types of disease and infirmity.

Today many young Chinese think that the "Eight Strands of the Brocade" are merely a number of specialised breathing exercises, whereas the name properly refers to the complete Chinese health arts. The vast majority of people are completely unaware of what a wide range these arts cover, and how many of them there are. One of the more specialised sections, and one of the most well known is Acupuncture (Hsia Chen Pien), which, along with all the other arts is still being carried on by dedicated Chinese, both inside and outside of China. Since the Chinese Revolution, China has come to enjoy the best of two worlds, the very old and the new: the ancient inheritance has been studied with greater enthusiasm than ever before, and together with modern medical science which has since been introduced, China has shown everyone another perfect example of the balance of the Yin and Yang.

"The Eight Strands of the Brocade" actually comprise eight distinct parts of the health arts, as follows:

1 Chen Tuan – Diagnosis.
2 Ch'ang Ming – Natural Health Therapy.
3 Ts'ao Yao – Herbal Therapy.
4 Wen Chiech'u – Contact Thermogenesis.
5 Hsia Chen Pien – Acupuncture.
6 Tien An – Spot Pressing.
7 T'ui Na – Massage.
8 Ch'ili Nung – The Way of Occlusion.

All these arts have been carried on by the Taoists through thousands of years. To further their knowledge they used themselves as guinea pigs, living and dying for the cause in which they believed, which had two main objectives: (1) maintaining a longer life on earth and (2) achieving a stronger spiritual link with the Supreme Spirit. In this they have aimed to abide by the laws of the universe, and accepting each day as it comes along, and becoming more conscious, aware and understanding that the organs of the body, the mind, physical strength and spiritual advancement all depend upon the amount of energy that is absorbed and stored within the human framework.

One source of such energy is through the food that is consumed, a second consists of correct breathing, and the third is the natural energy of the universe, "macrocosmic energy" (Ching Sheng Li). Macrocosmic energy is supplied free to all mankind, so that all may enjoy constant good health. All plants, bushes and trees depend on this same energy, as well as on the energy that they produce themselves; and the lack of it, or a restricted intake, can so weaken them that they wither and die. Human beings are affected in exactly the same way.

In ancient times men thrived by eating natural grown foods, uncontaminated by chemicals and pollution, and not only increased their knowledge of man's physical potential, but also became more spiritually aware. In those days, great philosophers, sages and spiritual leaders appeared, and many of the world's chief religions came into being. The teachings of men such as the Yellow Emperor, Lao Tzu, Chuang Tzu, Moses, Jesus Christ, Mohammed and Buddha were originally based on the natural laws of the universe, but unfortunately other men have misinterpreted these teachings, obscured them by adding ritual and attire, and introduced numerous laws to compel attendance at churches and temples. In this way the original teachings have often been lost, distorted or destroyed, and there are few teachers and preachers today who have any real depth of spiritual understanding. Words, themselves often representing a later, weakened form of the original teaching, are recited with little care for their meaning, and few teachers live as close to the spiritual world as they should if they are to set a good example for others. Thus it is that religion has become remote and out of touch, so fewer people now attend the services or say their prayers.

Many people are under the impression that the physical side of our lives is separate from our spiritual life, but this is not true, for the two sides represent the Yin and Yang aspects of our personal life, and therefore to strengthen one side one must also strengthen the other, so that eventually the two become as one, working as separate entities yet harmonise together as one working unit. What affects one will have its repercussion on the other. This is the true foundation of the Yin and Yang within ourselves, and they represent the Dual Monism, the combined unity and diversity, of our personal life, and the abiding law of living properly and correctly. (The Yin and Yang principles are discussed in greater detail in Chapter 2.)

Why is it, then, that all the great philosophers, sages and spiritual leaders appeared in approximately the same period way back in the past, yet there are none in this present day and age. There is a greater need of them now, as aggression, violence, murder and rape become more prevalent, so by cultivating the spiritual side of one's life, all these can be eradicated. So these great teachers illustrated to the world, that by living close to the earth, eating natural food without contamination from chemicals, polluted air and fluoridated waters, they become spiritually stronger.

In ancient China and in many other countries, the great teachers and philosophers were also healers in their own right, and had a deep understanding of the two sides of man, the physical and the spiritual. Through their dedication they developed great insight, perception, awareness and understanding of the laws of the universe, appreciated the utilisation of its dynamic energies and the reasons for the continual changes that take place.

Thanks to the early teachings of the "Sons of Reflected Light", China has led the field in this respect. The healer was paid by his patients only while they were well and so able to earn a living; but if they fell ill, and therefore had no income they paid him nothing. To the westerner this may seem a strange arrangement—but to the Chinese doctor there was a logical answer. Behind this lay the recognition that food including herbs was the best medicine, and that what nature provided free it was wrong to charge for.

That is the reason why, round about 3,000 BC, the Chinese laid down the five levels of physician who healed the spirit, conformed to the laws of nature, understood the universal energies, knew the human and animal bodies.

1. The Sage was the supreme doctor because he healed the spirit, and because of his experience he was able to point the way, externally and internally.
2. The next highest was the food doctor, who also administered herbal therapy, because both of these were closely linked to the laws of nature.
3. The third in line was the doctors of general medicine which includes acupuncture, spot pressing, massage, vibration healing and thermogenesis.
4. Fourth was the surgeon whose job it was to mend broken bones and internal fractures.
5. The animal doctors took the last place.

In all these aspects of healing the Chinese worked on the theory of the balance of the Yin and Yang, but the Taoists went one better, for they not only tried to harmonise the Yin and Yang within the human body, but also applied the same equilibrium to the spiritual side of their lives, through the soul and the spirit.

Their great endeavours and the enormous sacrifices they made bore fruit, and their work is still being carried on. Those of us who are involved in this are very proud of the fact, and we sincerely hope that we are keeping to the original teachings of the "Sons of Reflected Light", to whom we owe a great debt for showing us the way and for laying down the foundations on which our Chinese arts are built.

The Tao (Way) certainly has many features that we cannot always understand, but it is sure and positive. May we have our eyes opened so that we can see the true Way and follow it, according to the divine rules of the universe.

Chapter 1

The Tao

The Tao, the ordained Way of the entire cosmos, is not the complex, mystical concept that so many Western people believe or make it out to be. The truth is, that those who believe Taoism to be a mystical religion are not Taoists themselves, and do not realise that the Tao is the one way, that its course is unchangeable, and that its only function is to fulfil the divine will of the Supreme Spirit, or God. It affects all living matter—vegetation, animals and human beings—at all times, every second of every minute, through the time span of your present life, and your future lives to come.

It encompasses heaven, and the entire universe including our Earth planet, in all of the five directions within the full expanse of the entire firmament. Its efficiency is beyond normal human comprehension, and it creates and maintains the harmony between heaven and earth, according to the simple rules laid down by the Supreme Spirit.

In the very beginning it created order from chaos, with everything in its rightful place, and endowed it with the perfect balance of two influences, the Yin and the Yang, which form an integral part of everything. So from the one Tao came two principles which determine the stability of all creation, and control all the processes of evolution and changes taking place within it.

Though the Tao and its Yin and Yang constituents fill heaven and earth, they cannot be seen by the normal eye, yet are visible to the mind, soul and spirit. They are insubstantial yet are a composite substance of the material and the immaterial; they yield to change but are themselves absolute; their power is beyond normal human comprehension and yet their gentleness is softer than the air that touches the face. They are internal and external, microcosmic and macrocosmic, passive and active simultaneously linking through their contermination. They are completely individual, yet at the same time they are an harmonious part of each other—this has created Dual Monism, the combined unity and diversity of the cosmos.

Most people take the natural order of the Tao for granted, never giving it a second thought. That night follows day, spring follows winter, and so on, without change, is accepted without thought or question. Yet in accepting the natural order of the universe in this way, one is in fact recognising and accepting the Tao, albeit unconsciously. How natural and sensible it is, then, to live in accordance with the established order of nature, on which we all depend.

Therefore as we all rely on the normal manifestations of nature, which is absolutely dependent on the immutable ramifications of the universe, then the most sensible thing to do is to learn to follow the Tao. If you do made a full adjustment in your life, so as to keep to these natural laws, then your life will become serene and purposeful, your mental strength invincible, happiness will surround you, and life will then have a true meaning.

Once you have taken the initial step of looking outward, away from yourself, and recognising the work of the Tao, you will begin to see that the Tao is in control of everything, every minute of every day, and begin to recognise, understand and appreciate the reasons for it. To reach this understanding is not easy, for there may be many things that at first glance may seem wrong, or inexplicable, or even contrary to your trend of thought, and you may therefore become perplexed. However, you must learn to persevere and accept it, in the same way that you acknowledge the winds that blow, the waters that flow, and the clouds that hurry across the sky, then slowly through your own concentration you will gain mental and spiritual strength, you will harmonise with all things in the universe, and understanding will come, as surely as summer follows spring.

You will also need to look very closely at yourself. It is so easy to recognise the faults and good points of others, yet tend not to look very closely at the way we do things ourselves, our attitudes towards life and to others, our ambitions, our egos, and sometimes our infuriating habits which are apt to upset others, although we are often too blind to see it.

The Tao has created all the universe but does not boast about it; it leads everything along its own predestined and ordained way, yet you cannot see the controlling hand, though you can see the results. You were born and you will die—accept it! You were born with nothing and you will die with nothing—accept it!

Whether you are rich or poor, accept your path in life, don't boast or complain about it. Accept what is inevitable, and, once you recognise the Tao in your own life, then, and only then, will you see the changes that take place. Don't boast of your position or your wealth, for to do so could turn that Yang situation into a Yin one, for what was given can just as easily be taken away. Learn to control your thoughts by accepting everything as it comes along, and don't fret or worry about it. Don't plan ahead, for the Tao has already planned your future for you, and it is unchangeable. Have the strength and determination to see yourself through the rough or Yin patches, without moans or groans, without blaming others, and without self-pity; be happy to wait patiently for the Yang that is to come.

Above all, think of others, and learn to help and serve them at every opportunity, and great internal satisfaction will be derived, and happiness will abound constantly. This will also aid your mental and spiritual growth.

By getting closer to nature you can get closer to the Supreme Spirit, and become more receptive and perceptive of the Tao. So start on your Ch'ang Ming (Taoist Long Life) diet immediately and start to become healthier and physically stronger, for this will help to strengthen the mind and the spiritual side of your life, and enable you to gain a new dimension in other fields and influences within the realms of the universe.

Join the millions who follow the Taoist natural way of living, but it will take dedication and self discipline, but this is just another way of learning to control and understand yourself, and no longer eat out of habit. Your mind is in charge of your physical body, what you eat, drink, think and do is your own business, make a start now and ignore the sarcasm of those who think themselves wiser, though really ignorant. The man who lives with his head in the clouds cannot see the goodness under his feet.

Chapter 2

Yin and Yang

To many in the West the Yin and the Yang concept which was outlined by the Taoists, seems to create considerable contradictions and even a very extensive range of interpretations. Some claim to have studied the concept in great detail but tend to oppose others who claim the same. The fact is, however, that these people are not Taoists or otherwise they would understand the extreme simplicity of two dynamic yet gentle forces opposing or harmonising with one another. They are akin to an atheist talking about Christianity or man trying to explain how a fish feels. As such they see only the view from their window but fail to see the force that created what they see. They read the words, but do not appreciate the energy that was used to express them.

We are ONE with the Supreme Spirit but at the same time we still remain individuals, so through a natural principle a duality has automatically been created. This duality also applies to everything within the universe: just as every question can have two answers, a negative and positive. Everything has two sides, but remember too that each must have two halves, and that each of the halves has a top and a bottom, and that each of these has a back and a front, and so on and so on. Everything is one within itself, but at the same time it contains both Yin and Yang elements: being one it is monoism, but because of the diversity created by the universe, it has the balance of two—the Yin and Yang—which is therefore dualism. Therefore Dual Monoism covers the whole as well as the singular.

Such is the simplicity and yet complexity of the universe, but by appreciating and understanding the aspects of every single object, you will automatically obtain the double view of everything.

It cannot be stressed too often that Taoism is not a mystical religion, in fact it is not a religion at all; it is a belief and an understanding of the way that is ordained for everything in the universe. Mysticism and supposition had no place within Taoist thought, for they gained their scientific appreciation of cosmogony from the very source of creation—the Supreme Spirit—who educated them in the various differentials of force and energy, and showed them how these are available to everyone in the world through their physical, mental and spiritual spheres of the human body. So it is, even to this day, where true Taoism is being taught, these foundations, which were laid down by the Sages of ancient China thousands of years ago, are still being reinforced by millions through consciousness, awareness and understanding.

Taoism is quite simply a way of living according to the natural laws of the universe as created by the Supreme Spirit. The modern man-in-a-hurry, if he pauses long enough to think about it, will find that the answers to all problems of living were known to the early Taoists, and are readily available to all those who follow in the same path. The Taoist learns to work in constant harmony with nature every single day of his life, and, when the universe is fully understood, then there are no mysteries at all. All those who wish to progress will find that they need to pause and look backward first, so that they can begin to comprehend the laws of the Tao that control and activate everything within nature, including the complementary forces and dynamic energies that pervade it.

One example of the accuracy of the observations and calculations of the early Taoists, and thus of their understanding of the cosmos, is the yearly calendar that they devised. So accurate is it that it requires adjustment only every sixty years, instead of, as in the West, every four.

Before the world came into existence, there was the void, and in it the dynamic energy known as Ching Sheng Li or macrocosmic energy At the great inception, this force divided under strict control, into two parts, which came to be known to the Chinese as the Yin and the Yang. It was after this division that energy became substance, and heaven and earth became reality.

Characteristically Yin represents femininity, body, soul, earth, moon, night, water, cold, darkness, contraction, centripetal motion and a tendency to flow downwards. Yang, on the other hand, has opposite characteristics and some of these are masculinity, mind, spirit, heaven, sun, day, fire, heat, daylight, expansion, centrifugal motion and an upward direction of flow. Nothing, however, is wholly Yang or Yin, for where the one is present there is bound to be at least a small part of the other. What must be borne in mind is the fact that everything in nature has a constantly changing metabolism regulated by the Yin and Yang, and this includes our own bodies.

Since fire, heat and the sun are basically Yang, therefore the equator is the most Yang place on earth, and if you should travel away to the other extremes, to the north and south poles, where water is abundant, and cold and darkness are prevalent for six months of the year, then you are in the most Yin areas. However, most of the plants and fruits that grow in hot, Yang climates such as mangoes, oranges, pineapples contain a lot of water, which is Yin, whereas most fruits and roots in the colder Yin areas, are mainly Yang for they are smaller, contain more edible tissues and much less fluid.

Spring and summer along with wind and heat are Yang, while autumn and winter along with dryness and cold are Yin. Dryness can occur in a hot summer, so providing a Yin influence in a Yang season. This is another example of the duality of nature.

This duality is also evident in the human body, for the viscera are Yin whilst the bowel system is Yang; the exterior of the body is Yang and the interior is Yin; the right side of the body is Yang and the left side is Yin; and so on. There is no escaping these simple yet natural laws within ourselves, and it must be fully appreciated that to attain true harmony then means must be found to achieve the correct balance at all times.

It is within our own power to see that this is so, and to understand that any change in this balance could alter our physical, mental and spiritual situations. Therefore to correct any deterioration we must be prepared to change to a Ch'ang Ming health diet, alter our way of life, our attitudes and code of conduct to others, and in extreme cases of necessity, such as a serious illness, we may even have to change our environment.

We have no one to blame but ourselves if we upset the balance of the Yin and Yang and become ill, or suffer from any sickness, for we have created our own deterioration and must therefore accept the consequences, and not blame others for our own mistake or carelessness.

Make a start now by changing your own life for the better, by reading this book carefully, and diligently adhering to its recommendations, then you can obtain an excellent internal balance, and so open the way to permanent good health and a happier and more rewarding existence. Once you have started you will be pleasantly surprised how simple it all is, and this should encourage you to persevere even more and thereby deepen your understanding of the Taoist arts.

By being ill at any time then this is an obvious sign that you have upset the balance within your body and are therefore now Yin, but changing your eating habits and becoming healthier again you have corrected the balance and have turned it into Yang. This should show you how two different conditions can be brought into balance—affecting one person—You.

Chapter 3

The Five Elements

The "Five Elements" (Wu Hsing) are of fundamental importance to the Chinese arts, and many volumes have been written about them to try and explain the intrinsicality of this Taoist concept. However, while these may be helpful in putting forward the basic theories, only the practice of living in full accordance with these laws of the universe can give you the full appreciation and true understanding of the importance of the "Five Elements".

In the previous chapters we have seen the close relationship between the Tao and the Yin and Yang, and it was from these that the "Five Elements" came into being, through the reciprocal interaction between heaven and earth. Whilst we may not realise it, the "Five Elements" play an important part in our daily lives, for they beset us in every conceivable way, through our emotions, our thoughts, our actions, the food and drink that we consume, our health, and the strength and growth of our spiritual life. In addition, they can influence our lives through seasonal changes, climatic fluctuations and the time of the day or night. All this was fully understood by the ancient sages of China who appreciated the basic principles of the Tao, the founder of all things.

They also understood the harmony or opposition that each object has with all other things in the universe, and it gave them, as a result, a very deep insight into the workings of the human body, and how to diagnose sickness through the pulses, and through touch, visual observation, speech and smell, and through the intuition and experience that only time and a deep understanding can bring.

The "Five Elements" are Wood, Fire, Soil, Metal and Water, which in turn represent the five forces of energy, or the five sections of change that exist within everything in the universe. They are all an integral part of the Yin and Yang, and the Yin and Yang is within each of them, making for an overall harmonious balance, which is the Tao.

The theory underlying this ancient trend of thought is fully expressed in the Yellow Emperor's Classic of the Nei Ching (Internal Health), and proves without doubt that anything that has a beginning also has an end; and that the end is the commencement of something new, and that from a maximum point there must be a decline to a minimum level, and vice versa. This constant change is the natural order of all things, according to the fundamental laws of the Tao. Despite what modern scientists may say, these laws are just as valid today as they were when they were first formulated, and they are still being used successfully in Chinese medicine and treatment.

The harmony between the elements is quite simple when you consider that they exist through a unique relationship to one another. The ancients put it thus: *wood* is food for the *fire*, and when the fire dies down all that is left is ashes which eventually become part of the *soil*, in which the *metals* and other minerals are formed, and when these are melted down they turn into *water*, which nourishes the trees, which give us *wood*, and so each has helped the other not only to become established in the first place, but through their constant endeavours they each supply the essential for the other to survive.

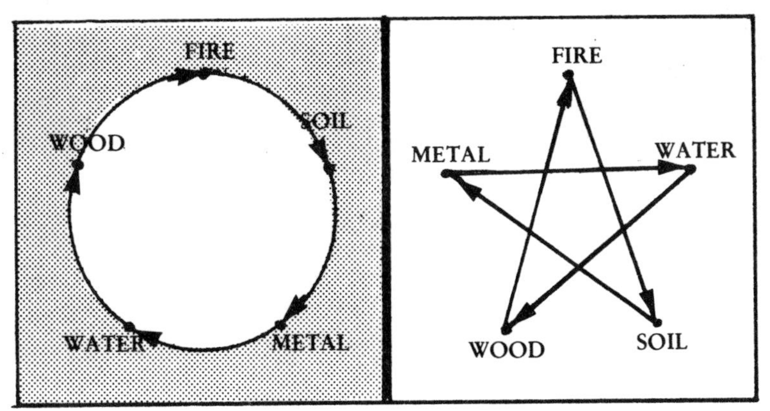

The Harmony of the Five Elements

However, the elements can oppose and thereby destroy each other: *metal* can cut wood into shreds, *wood* can penetrate into the soil, *soil* can stop the flow of water, *water* can extinguish fire, and the heat of *fire* can dissolve metal.

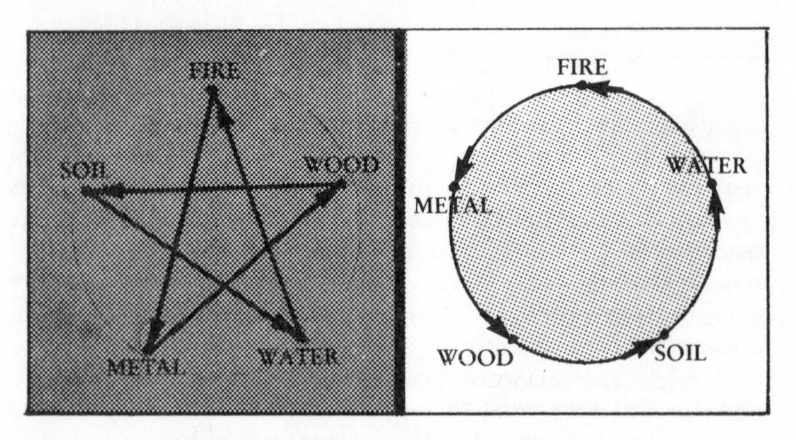

The Opposition of the Five Elements

The number five refers not only to the number of elements, but also to many other related groups. The table overleaf shows how these fit into the Yin and Yang equations of the Tao. Man and everything about him either harmonises with or opposes nature. So long as he is in harmony with the universal laws, he flourishes, but, if he goes against them, his health and everything else about him suffers.

Therefore, an understanding of those laws is essential if man is to live a happy, healthy and long life, and that is exactly what Ch'ang Ming is all about and why the Taoists went so thoroughly into every aspect of the physical, mental and spiritual spheres. For man is an integral part of the universe, or should be, for his body is under the control of the mind, and his mind is controlled by the soul, and the soul by the spirit. If his thoughts go haywire and are influenced or controlled by lust, ambition, jealousy or hate, he will close the channels to the spirit, and lose authority and the power to regulate his own body, with the result that its formation and accumulation of vital internal energy begins to fail, the whole system starts to decline, and illness follows.

As you can see from the "Five Elements" chart, if, for instance, you have a weakness in the lungs, the autumn is the season that should make you extremely wary, and the chest should be well protected, particularly when snow covers the ground and the air becomes dry. You will also find that you will have a tendency to cry, and this will mean more mucus secreted from the nose. This will make you feel low and your nervous system will suffer, for you will be continuously full of grief, and through it all you will find that you have trouble with your skin and your hair, both of which will feel dry and lifeless. You will be at your lowest ebb in the evening, and, whilst you will also suffer from back trouble, you will also find that you also have inconvenience from your large intestine. Under these conditions, the best food to eat is brown rice, and occasionally some peaches.

As regards the harmony between the five elements, you will notice that wood (liver) leads on to fire (heart), which in turn leads on to the soil (spleen), and so on, until the circle is complete. This rotation allows one organ to draw energy from another, for instance, the heart from the liver, and the spleen from the heart, and so on, and then to pass on any surplus vitality to the next organ in the cycle. This is a perfect example of the process of giving and taking within the realms of nature, and we could all learn a lesson from this by taking only as much as is necessary. However, if the body's energy levels become depleted, each organ will draw as much as it can from the other, until every organ is completely run down. This dramatic deterioration of the body can lead to many serious illnesses—cancer being one of them.

Let us look at it another way. The liver (wood) passes energy to the muscles, which in turn helps to make a strong heart. The heart (fire) gives nourishment to the blood and the arteries, and they in turn pass it on to the spleen (soil) which nurtures the flesh, and which gives added strength to the lungs. The lungs (metal) feed the skin and hair, and they continue the circle by giving the kidneys a boost. The kidneys (water) give food to the bones and nails, and their act of duty is to feed the liver. So from this you will fully appreciate that:

1 The liver is in charge of the muscles and tissues.
2 The heart is in charge of the arteries and the texture of the body.
3 The spleen is in charge of the flesh, including the lips.
4 The lungs are in charge of the skin and hair.
5 The kidneys are in charge of the bones and nails.

The Five Elements

	Greater Yang	Lesser Yang	Middle Yang/Yin	Lesser Yin	Greater Yin
Five Elements	Wood	Fire	Soil	Metal	Water
Viscera	Liver	Heart	Spleen and Pancreas	Lungs	Kidneys
Bowels	Gall Bladder	Small Intestine	Stomach	Large Intestine	Bladder
Seasons	Spring	Summer	Late Summer	Autumn	Winter
Daily Periods	Morning	Noon	Afternoon	Evening	Night
Planets	Jupiter	Mars	Saturn	Venus	Mercury
Directions	East	South	Equator	West	North
Weather	Dry/Crisp	Fog/Mist	Mellow	Snow	Frost/Ice
Colours	Green	Red	Yellow	White	Black
Climatic Conditions	Wind	Heat	Humidity	Dryness	Cold
Controlling influence	Spirit	Soul	Mind	Ambition	Physical strength
Creation	Inspiration	Aspiration	Intellect	Dominance	Will
Emotions	Shouting	Laughing	Singing	Weeping	Groaning
Fluids	Tears	Sweat	Saliva	Mucus	Urine

Anatomy – externally	Tissues	Complexion	Lips	Hair	Nails
Senses	Sight	Hearing	Taste	Smell	Touch
Openings	Eyes	Ears	Mouth	Nose	Lower Cavities
Mental stress	Anger	Joy	Sympathy	Grief	Fear
Sickness	Nerves	Viscera	Tongue	Back	Cavities
Best treatment	Spiritual cure	Ch'ang Ming	Herbal therapy	Acupuncture	Thermogenesis
Ideal Food	Wheat	Corn	Millet	Rice	Peas, Beans
Vegetables	Leeks	Shallots	Mallow	Onions	Coarse Greens
Fruit	Apples	Strawberry Cherry	Dates Olives	Peaches Melons	Grapefruit Oranges
Animal Foods	Pheasants Egg yolks	Turkey Pigeon	Chicken	Rabbit Hares	Pork Beef
Dairy foods	Goat's milk	Vegetarian Cheese	Edam Cheese	Milk	Yoghurt Butter
Drinks and herbs	Jinseng	Mugwort Fo Ti Tien	Thyme	Fruit Juices Beer	Coffee Tea
Liking for	Sour	Bitter	Sweet	Pungent	Salty
Avoid food that is	Rancid	Overdone	Fragrant	Rotten	Putrid

The five flavours, sour, bitter, sweet, pungent and salty, are all said to have certain intimate powers which they influence at certain times of the year, but only to particular parts of the body with whom they have harmony. This also applies to people suffering from specific weaknesses or sickness, for they should, in certain seasons, be especially careful where they travel. Someone suffering from kidney or bladder trouble, for instance, would be unwise venturing north in winter where there could be hard frost and ice, and where the atmosphere is colder. He should follow the line of harmony best suited to his physical weakness (i.e. travel east) or wait to enjoy the air of spring.

The chart shows each organ and element is related to a specific colour, which is extremely important in the arts of diagnosis. For wood the colour is green, fire is red, soil is yellow, for metal white, and for water it is black. Green is closely related to blue, for due to refraction of light one could take on the tone of the other, so although the ancients of China have specified green, remember it can refer to both.

If anyone has a too red a complexion, this can indicate heart problems or stress, while green or bluish tints can show that the liver is in trouble and needs attention. Yellow is related to the spleen and pancreas and is an indicator of jaundice, and a pale whitish skin signifies bad lungs. Take a look at the number of people in the street that have this look—all of them prey to colds, sinus troubles, asthma and influenza. Black or dark brown indicates kidney complaints.

Anyone suffering from kidney trouble should be extremely wary of the cold (especially the cold night air) and make sure that he is well wrapped up all the time. His diet should include peas, beans and coarse greens, the latter will also include Chinese cabbage (Pai Tsai), and he should carefully watch the colour of his urine, for this is an indicator of the process of internal change.

The five viscera are the Yin organs of the body while the five bowel systems are the Yang organs. When only one organ has a weakness, this can be tackled in a straightforward manner (for instance, if the trouble is the heart, which is Yin, this can be dealt with through Yang foods and herbs). In other words, one kind of illness in an organ can be countered by the opposite influence.

However, as the Nei Ching points out, if there are two Yin organs affected, then one Yang influence will not be enough to balance the good and the bad, so further steps have to be taken. This is where a thorough understanding of the harmony and opposition of the "Five Elements" is so essential to appreciate the depth of the Chinese arts in relation to the human body.

If an illness is retained over a long period, then gradually all the organs become affected. The five Yin viscera multiplied by the "Five Elements" gives twenty-five types of disharmony, and if the illness becomes still worse, so that the Yin organs start drawing off energy from the five Yang bowel systems (again, five times five, equals twenty-five, types of disharmony), then the number of points of opposition becomes astronomical, for twenty-five multiplied by twenty-five is 625. When there are that many things wrong with the body, the situation is frightening; this is what the advanced cancer cases are going through.

Thus, with any illness, it is vital to treat it as early as possible; or even better still, get advice from your nearest Ch'ang Ming consultant, so that he can put you on the right lines before an illness can develop. In other words, cure it before it happens, for this is the best way of preventing illness; for it will give you unbroken and constant good health.

Chapter 4

Time and Energy

We now have a greater insight to the Tao, the Yin and Yang, the five elements, but the ancient history of the Taoists has also given us two other aspects of the Chinese use of numerology. The use of numbers has played a great part in all aspects of life for the Chinese, for it is a very easy way to relate to things and to make comparisons. From one (the Tao) came two (the Yin and Yang), from two came five (the Five Elements), and from five came the multitude of 10,000 things that exist on earth and within the universe. In this chapter, some more aspects of Chinese numerology will be outlined, as part of a discussion of time and energy.

Within 200 years there are going to be great changes in this world of ours, for time and energy are slowly moving into a flux of alteration. This could lead to China becoming the number-one nation of the world, and to women becoming the leaders in all professions and in politics, and already minor changes are beginning to resolve themselves. Whatever the future may hold, however, nothing can stop the fulfilment of the Tao, so learn to accept the inevitable. If you do then life will go smoothly for you; but fight it and you will become bad tempered and aggressive and change to a Yin life, which will be really tough for you, for you cannot fight the universal laws, neither can you fight the Supreme Spirit, not can you expect to alter the path that has been spiritually laid down for you. Try and resist the inevitable and you will lose precious time and energy.

Time is extremely important to us, for it never stands still and we must make the best use of it and utilise every minute for energy is necessary for us, not only to survive, but that we may live long and enjoy constant good health. The ancient Chinese found that the development of woman and man could be explained in terms of seven and eight year cycles, and although it was formulated on the growth of people in China at the time, and since then things have altered as living standards in various countries have changed, the patterns are still recognisable.

The development of Woman

At birth she is Yin.
At seven her teeth and hair have quite noticeable growth.
At fourteen she starts to menstruate, and can therefore bear children.
At twenty-one she is fully developed, and is at her best.
At twenty-eight her body is firm and flourishing.
At thirty-five her face begins to wrinkle and she starts to lose hair.
At forty-two her hair starts to turn grey and her arteries begin to harden.
At forty-nine her menstruation ceases, and she can no longer bear children.
At fifty-six her hair turns white and her activity becomes less.
At sixty-three she starts to turn Yang mentally.

The development of Man

He is born Yang.
At eight he loses his baby teeth.
At sixteen he starts to secrete semen.
At twenty-four he is fully grown.
At thirty-two his muscles are hard and firm.
At forty his sexuality weakens and he starts to lose hair.
At forty-eight his teeth start to decay and his skin wrinkles.
At fifty-six his hair turns grey and his testes diminish.
At sixty-four he starts to turn mentally Yin.

Why and how these progressions were originally formulated no one seems to know, but the Taoists, because of their closeness to the spiritual world, believe that they were founded on the spiritual growth and advancement of each individual.

The numbers seven and eight crop up in other connexions as well, for instance, women, being spiritually stronger than man, reincarnates only seven times on average, while man usually reincarnates at least eight times. This is related to the seven planes to heaven, which is the control centre of the universe, and the home of the Supreme Spirit. The planes are as follows:

1 Heaven.
2 Celestial orbit.
3 Astral plain.
4 Stratosphere.
5 Magnetic belt.
6 Atmospheric field.
7 Earth.

The eighth is accounted for by man's extra "shift" on earth, and beyond the final reincarnation there is no sex discrimination: all are spirits, and all are One with the Supreme Spirit, and, because they are without egoism, ambition, or emotions, follow the Tao exactly according to the wishes of the Master.

The seven or eight stages to heaven, including our spiritual advancement which we develop here on earth, cover the complete development of our entire spiritual lives, and the Taoists knew that the first step towards the ultimate objective (which has been referred to as spiritual alchemy), is to start work now. It is not by coincidence, luck or chance that this book came into your hands, nor is it a fluke that you are finding the time to read it—it was meant to be. Therefore don't waste the rest of your years in this present life-span on earth, but open your mind and try to follow the path that is being pointed out to you, and you will find a world, within this world that we live in, that you never before realised existed.

Once you have started to develop on the right lines, remember to go step by step in easy stages, for your spiritual growth cannot be hurried or accelerated. The growth and expansion of your physical self in harmony with your mind, soul and spirit can put you on the right path, even though you may not, at the present time, have any thoughts about the spiritual side of your life. Be that as it may, always remember that the type of apprenticeship that you serve in this life is the foundation on which you build in your next life.

Closeness to nature will bring you closer to the fundamental laws of the universe, so learning to eat and drink the Ch'ang Ming way will bring you back to the natural order of things. Your health will improve to a degree that will certainly surprise you, and, whilst all around you have colds and 'flu, you will be carrying on untouched. But constant good health is only one minor aspect of the full benefits that you will derive by following this sensible course, for in addition, you will feel more relaxed, your nerves will be more settled you will find that you are no longer so emotional and will be able to cope calmly with the ups and downs of your daily life, which will begin to take on a new meaning for you. You will see things that you overlooked before, and you will open a new phase in your life, and at last you will fully understand what happiness, coupled with good health, really means. Through the good health of the body, new channels in the mind will be opened up, your energy levels will rise, and so your vitality and spiritual awareness will increase. You will experience greater harmony in every direction.

To help the spiritual side of your life, learn to think good and do good whenever you can, never let a bad thought enter the mind, and by so doing, you will learn to control your thoughts, emotions and actions at all times. Never harass, harm or hurt anyone, either by thought or by deed, no matter what they do or do not. Everyone has his own path in life, which he follows in his own way and at his own speed. What may be suitable to you, may not be suitable for someone else.

As you progress and change, it may seem to you that the world has completely altered. It hasn't—only you have; and this change will stand you in good stead not only in the future years of your present life, but also—though you may not believe it—in your future lives.

One of the many improvements will be in the amount of energy at your disposal. There are in fact four distinct types of energy in the human body, the physical, mental, internal and external, and each one has various sub-divisions.

You use the physical energy every day of your life, whether you are at work, at play or even when you relax, and invariably few people know very little about it or how it is acquired, for we are all apt to take it for granted and never give it a passing thought. It does not, however, depend on big muscles, in fact, in most cases it is completely the opposite, for tense muscular systems generally retard the natural expansion of your physical vitality. That is why the best way to advance it is through the exercises of T'ai Chi Ch'uan (Supreme Ultimate), K'ai Men (Taoist Yoga) and the very soft style of Chinese Boxing (Kungfu) known as Feng Shou (Hand of the Wind). These render the muscles and ligaments gentle suppleness and flexibility and make the old feel young and enable the young to feel really dynamic

Of course, Ch'ang Ming is the essential counterpart to attain this goal, through such exercises, for it purifies the organs, increases the goodness in the bloodstream, and improves the circulation, so enabling any weaknesses in the metabolism to be overcome and physical vitality to be increased to the maximum, thereby enabling you to grow old without being old.

Mental energies are also a part of your daily life. You use them for thinking, activating your body, and restoring vitality which may have been depleted through worry, emotions, stress and strain. Mental energies may also be used to explore the innermost depths of the self, through hypersensitivity, sensory perception, concentrated control of the internal and external energies, and the various fields of meditation, which in Taoism has many sections.

Complete and utter relaxation of the mind, body and spirit is essential for personal well-being and Ch'ang Ming is the first key to this. By its means the various energy channels can be thrown open, so that the energies flow freely; but, so that they are not wasted, the mind must be in complete control all the time, so that the energy channels can be closed when required.

To gain, retain, store and recharge mental energy to the best advantage requires a healthy (but not necessarily a physically fit) body, strong internal energy, and the development of the external force. Whilst the energies all operate separately and are distinct from each other, they are interdependent and can be harmonised to become one, when required.

Internal energy (Nei Pu Chi) also called microcosmic energy and the Vitality power (Sheng Chi) is an internal part of every human being, and something that everyone is born with, though from the age of about five or six years, you start to use your physical strength more and more, and therefore your internal energy becomes dormant and declines. Its benefit to the human body is colossal, for it helps to fight bacteria within the bloodstream and protects the body against disease.

It is invisible to the human eye, although its effects are visible; it has no aroma; you cannot hear it; and the whole of your natural life is centred around it. If it is weakened, you are prey to numerous illnesses, and if you lack it you are at risk from cancer, hypothermia and many other cold sicknesses. Internal energy is heat and generates heat, and so may be likened to a system of storage heating: when it is not needed, it is stored up for future use. It is important that it should not be wasted, or it will not be available when the health of the body really needs it.

There are only two ways in which internal energy can be built up and maintained at a reasonable level within the body: by eating and drinking the Ch'ang Ming way, and by regular deep-breathing exercises through the lower abdomen (Tan T'ien).

External or macrocosmic energy (Ching Sheng Li) comes down from heaven, passes through all things, even our own bodies, goes into the earth, and in so doing gathers further energy and vitality, then goes back to heaven again, and in so doing it passes through many other things. It is everywhere, and passes through you constantly whether you are awake or asleep, and is doing so even as you read this. However, if you remain constantly indoors, then your share of it is reduced by the walls, ceiling, and things around you; so, whenever you can, get out into the fresh air, for this will help to revitalise you.

The early Taoists learned through their infinite search for spiritual alchemy to harness, store, control and use external energy, and it is this that enables many of them to live to 150 to 200 years of age. You can too, if you join us in the knowledge that age is only the number of earth years, and that at sixty or more you have the skin, mind, energy and vitality that you had when you were only twelve years of age. Time is nothing; it is how you use it, live it and utilise it that really matters, and your spiritual growth depends upon it.

Out of all the energies that we have or should have, external energy is the most important, for it was this that brought the universe into being, and created all plant life, fish, mammals, animals and ourselves. We too are animals, but what separates them from humanity is not the power of the brain, but that we possess a spirit, which is composed of the same energy.

The Taoists realised this fact thousands of years ago, and knew that the development of this energy was essential to the spiritual life, for it is external energy that enables the spirit to be reincarnated and that when you die ensures that your spirit has the vitality to return to the astral plains where it will rest, until the next time round. It was this energy that enabled Jesus Christ to rise from the dead and go to heaven, and this is exactly what happens to your own spirit.

External energy is also of great value in healing. It is indeed truly wonderful that the energy that gives us life also enables us to give life to others, so proving again the harmony of the universe.

Chapter 5

Traditional Chinese Diagnosis

In the West when a person becomes ill he goes to the doctor, who seeks to classify the symptoms into a specific group and thereby form an opinion and give his diagnosis. Chinese traditional doctors however, do not have to wait until a person becomes ill or depend on the symptoms, for they are trained in the basic principles of the Yin and Yang and can thereby diagnose a weakness or illness before it is fully apparent, and, in many cases, even before the person concerned is aware that there is something wrong. It is the Chinese physician's meticulous training in the "Eight Classifications" (Pa Fen Lei) and the "Five Systems of Examination" (Wu Chen Ch'a) that enables him to do this, for over thousands of years these methods have proved very successful and extremely efficient.

The Eight Classifications are as follows:

1 Yin	2 Yang
3 Internal.	4 External
5 Cold.	6 Hot
7 Decreased levels.	8 Increased levels.

Through an appreciation and understanding of all these groups, and the fusing of all the information obtained into one conclusion a full diagnosis of the patient's condition, from the head to the toes, and from the innermost depths of the body to the external symptoms, can be concluded.

In the West, the classification of illness is a complex business, for they give every ailment or sickness a different name, some of which are almost unpronounceable. In China, by contrast, we recognise only two categories of illness, and they are either Yin or Yang. It is as simple as that, for these two principles are basic to everything in the universe, including illness.

Illness is made by man, and caused by the restriction of internal energy, which is Yin, and which is the harmonious counterpart of external energy which is Yang. If the body, mind and the spirit are truly healthy, then man can live his whole life without catching the slightest illness, not even the common cold; but, if he disturbs the proper functions of the body, then he becomes Yin, and this contraction will severely hamper the flow of energies which are so necessary for good health. If, however, the passage of internal and external energies through the body is allowed to flow completely unchecked, then the body will suffer the consequences of over-activity, and this expansion will produce a Yang illness.

The first question to be asked about a weakness or an illness is, then, whether it is Yin or Yang, internal or external, and if it is caused by a deterioration in the internal organs, or by external factors, such as the weather, seasonal changes, or some transgression of the laws of the universe.

Within the Eight Classifications all the odd numbers represent the Yin aspects. As already noted, the earth, internal energy, contraction, darkness, cold, water, and so on are basically Yin. So too is turbulence in the earth's atmosphere (Yin), which causes clouds (Yang) to form in the sky; the pressure of external cosmic energy (Yang) on those clouds has a tendency to create a too Yang situation, and as a result rain (Yin) falls.

It is due to this interplay that can affect and influence each or both, that extreme cold (Yin) can cause feverish conditions (Yang) in the body. The person with a Yin illness may perspire on the outside yet feel cold inside; this is connected with the fact that the viscera are Yin. Generally, when a person is suffering from a Yin complaint, he not only feels cold, but also feels weak and lifeless, does not want to eat very much, feels very sorry for himself, and therefore wants to be alone.

The Yang aspects in the Eight Classifications are denoted by even numbers, and naturally, are the opposite of the Yin aspects. If, for instance, a person is suffering from intense heat internally, he will generally suffer from a damp hand, his skin will be cold, and he will break out in goose pimples. A person suffering from a Yang illness is generally lively, although his breathing could be heavy and laboured and may even at times be sporadic, and his breath could also have a distinct smell. Invariably he will have a coated or furred tongue, for the bowels systems are Yang.

The "Five Systems of Examination" (Wu Chen Ch'a) also conform to the basic principles of the Five Elements, and are related to the five senses of the human body, as follows:

1 Use of the *mouth* to ask questions about the illness and how long it has persisted; where and how often and at what times the pains are being felt; what hereditary tendencies are there in the family; what kind of work the patient does; any appetite problems; eating and drinking habits including the likes and dislikes; consumption of drugs and medicines; and so on.
2 Use of the *eyes* to observe the colour of the skin and complexion, the lines and contours of the flesh, the shape of the face, the angles of the nose and eyebrows, the shape and length of the nose and lips, veins on the hands, colour and size of the fingernails, height, weight, way of walking, and so forth.
3 Use of the *nose* to detect the smell of bad breath and any body odours.
4 Use of the *ears* to listen to the vibrations of the patient's body, the pitch of the voice, rumblings from the bowel system, any coughing, the patient's breathing, and so on.
5 Use of the *touch* through the hands and fingers which involves feeling all the pulses (Chen Mo), which is a complete art within itself; to feel lumps, bumps, swellings and other malformations; to carry out Spot Pressing (Tien Chen).

By means of the Five Systems and the Eight Classifications, the patient's energy level and its pattern can be fully assessed and any disturbances can be fully appreciated and understood. These disturbances fall into two areas, internal and external (Nos. 3 and 4 of the Eight Classifications), and they can also be interpreted as a movement—into two main directions—and which can be defined as:

1 Those that flow from inside to an outside point.
2 Those that flow from the outside to an inside area.

Those in the first group are generally caused by weaknesses in the constitution which will include those that may have been inherited at birth, and also those illnesses that become obvious after years and years of bad eating and drinking habits. Into the second group fall injuries of all kinds, external infections, and disturbances brought about by changes in atmospheric conditions caused by heat, cold or dampness.

All physicians in China know that the greater the contraction the greater the Yin influence; and the larger the expansion the stronger the Yang tendency. So it is that all things reflect these two polarities, for everything has its mirror image. What starts at the bottom will eventually find its way to the top, and that which begins on the inside must in time present itself on the outside, and the external will reflect and influence the internal.

Of course, it takes a long time to master all the many and varied aspects of the Five Systems of Examination, for it is only through experience that full understanding and the depth of the intuition is obtained. Constantly bear in mind the theory of the Five Elements, for all things are interrelated, and to arrive at a full diagnosis all the evidence that you accumulate through your senses must be taken into account. Not only will you have a very deep appreciation of everything that may go on inside or outside of your own body, but it will enable you to understand what others are going through, more and more, and eventually you will be able to help them because you understand their problems.

Chapter 6

Diagnosis by Observation

Everything in the universe came into existence in accordance with the wishes of the Tao, and conforms to the principles of the Yin and Yang. The intricate balance between the two is characterised by very definite visible signs, which in one form or another can be plainly seen on the body of every human being even where attempts are made to hide or disguise them through the use of powder, cream or other make-up.

Over the centuries, women and men have used enormous quantities of make-up to hide or disguise the pimples, colourings, wrinkles and scars indicative of bad health, past and present, yet, do not appreciate that all the make-up in the world cannot erase the signs of a person's bad health, and no surgery can eradicate the cause. Curiously enough, many characteristics that in the West are viewed or accepted as signs of beauty, really indicate bad health and extreme Yin tendencies.

For instance, a tall, thin body, big lips, thin eyebrows, long upcurling eyelashes, colouring around the eyes, a long thin nose, a long angular face, and swinging hips are all Yin characteristics and signs of bad health. If one recognises bad health as beauty, then one might as well look for beauty in rape, murder and in other forms of aggression, for these unhealthy signs are Yin too.

When you were in your mother's womb, you naturally received some of your parents' characteristics, together with some of their strengths and weaknesses. Some of them become manifest soon after birth, while others remain hidden and only show themselves at a later date, developing slowly over the years. All these things, including some that you may not yet be aware of or suspect, are outwardly expressed by your own body, from which your life history may be read, and it is so exposed that everyone who understands our arts can read it with ease. Whilst you might be able to hide some of it with your clothes or your make-up for some of the time, you cannot hide or disguise it all of the time.

The value of all this is the fact that you have one real consolation, for once you have recognised the weaknesses in your own system, and are able to read the history of your own life, you will be able to appreciate the biological fluctuations that constantly go on within your own body, and therefore be able to do something about them. Furthermore, if you become very practised at diagnosis by observation, you will be able to help others by identifying their own weaknesses, and perhaps by warning them of the beginnings of illnesses of which they have not been aware, they might be prepared to change their eating and drinking habits to overcome those weaknesses.

All sicknesses are man-made, and whilst there are many things that may aggravate a weakness in the body, man alone is responsible for his own vulnerability to illness for he has created the basic cause. Once you have faced this truth in your own case, then you can set about living to the universal laws of nature.

If you have been ill or are suffering an illness at present, don't be too critical of yourself, even though you know that you created it yourself; you were simply ignorant of the simple laws of nature, and the intricate workings of the universe, and so therefore can be excused for not knowing that if you had changed your eating and drinking habits earlier, then even the common cold would have been a thing of the past.

So no matter how ill you might feel at this moment, or even if you suffer no sickness whatsoever and feel on top of the world, now is the time to appraise the situation and face the simple facts of life, by the simple process of self diagnosis through the natural laws of the Yin and Yang, created by the Tao.

Diagnosis by Observation (Kuanch'a Chentuan) may sound as if you have to be a qualified scientist, but it is nothing of the kind and you will find it quite simple. All it requires is that you look closely and truthfully at yourself, and understand what your eyes can see. Do this now, as you read through the rest of this chapter, which asks you whether you are Yin or Yang, and for you to put yourself into one or the other category, through simply identifying the characteristics of each and matching them against yourself. Go on, go and get a mirror, have a good look at yourself, and jot down on a piece of paper each of your characteristics.

Are you Yin?

Skin Colours

White. This colour denotes diseases that are found in the skin and in the hair, and being Yin it also indicates that the person has poor blood and is suffering from anaemia.

A pasty white coloration, is an extremely common hue amongst people in the Western world, and there may appear white spots on the face or the body, all of which are caused by over-consumption of dairy products, such as milk, cheese, cream, butter, eggs and yoghurt.

A pallid transparent or glossy-looking skin generally denotes bad lungs. The skin is always chilly and cold to the touch, and the person is very sensitive to atmospheric conditions, especially damp or cold weather.

All the various shades of white skin are Yin, but the person with the pale or pallid coloured skin is more extremely Yin than any of the others, for it can also be an outward sign of such serious diseases as tuberculosis and leprosy, or it could denote that the person could be suffering from respiratory allergies, such as sinus trouble, hayfever and asthma.

Grey. This is another common colour amongst people in the West, and it reflects a hardening condition within the liver, making it a Yin complaint. The person having this colour has a natural tendency to become angry very quickly and easily, may flare up suddenly on the spur of the moment without apparent reason, and yet the same person can suffer periods of deep depression and shed tears unexpectedly.

Black. "Black" signifies a colour between dark brown and black. It indicates kidney problems, and is Yin, and points to an accumulation of waste matter in the bloodstream. This occurs when the kidneys are over-worked and thus unable to filter the blood properly. This toxic matter seeks an outlet and it rises slowly to the surface of the skin, causing discoloration, but more often it will be seen in the form of dark brown or black spots, known in the West as "beauty spots"! These spots are usually caused by very Yin drinks and foods, such as iced drinks (especially the synthetic and manufactured ones) and frozen foods, and also by drugs and strong medicaments. Sometimes the accumulation is so great at any one particular spot that a black mole is formed; and all this points to an excess consumption of meat and meat products. A person who has moles generally has a tendency to be mentally apprehensive.

Yellow. Yellow and even to a deeper hue of a light orange is a definite indication of problems connected with the spleen and pancreas and the liver. The colour can also show up in the whites of the eyes and it is connected with jaundice. The pancreas being one of the main organs controlling the amount of sugar in the body, then it can be understood that an excess consumption of sweets and sugar can create trouble in this organ.

Red. Red is normally a Yang colour. Sometimes it may appear all over the body, and sometimes it may appear only on certain parts of the anatomy, but don't put blushing into this category, as this is an active yet perfectly normal sign.

The gums should normally be pink in colour, but if they are red, then this shows that the blood capillaries have expanded, and it is a sure indication of a Yin intake mainly through drugs and medicines.

If the skin has patches of redness, is very dry and perhaps has a tendency to flake, and itches especially at night, this could be owing to jaundice or to an allergy, and it is advisable to stay away from seasoned and spicy foods, animal foods, and alcohol of all kinds.

If parts of the face become red during cold weather, it is an indication that the circulation is very poor, and that there is blood stagnation or an excess of blood. It is advisable to cut out all meat from the diet.

The Nei Ching explains that if someone is ill and is suffering from a bout of fever, then the part of the face that turns red indicates which organ is affected, and is a directive where treatment should be directed.

1 A red complexion indicates the heart.
2 A red nose shows sickness of the spleen.

3 Red on the left side of the jaw points to the liver being under duress.
4 Red on the right side of the jaw signifies disease in the lungs.
5 A red chin points to trouble in the kidneys.

In all these instances a very strong Yin influence is indicated and headaches, perspiration and even vomiting may be experienced.

Rosy red cheeks every afternoon, accompanied by sweaty hands and feet; with perhaps, profuse sweating during the night, a dry mouth and a red tongue, then it could be an indicator of tuberculosis. If you have these symptoms then get it checked straight away.

Don't, however, mistake the reddish glow on the skin of a new or very young baby as a bad sign, remember it has only just been born, and is therefore going through a Yang period as it starts to grow and expand. So for the infant it is a good healthy colour and is perfectly natural.

Other parts of the body may show signs of redness, but these will be dealt with in other sections.

Pink. Normally a pinkish skin is a sign of good health, but should anyone get a deep pink glow in the cheeks in the afternoon, this, together with the other symptoms mentioned above, could show a tendency towards tuberculosis.

Blue. Blue and purple colouring, especially in the veins and the capillaries which show through the tissues of the skin, is a Yin complaint, and indicates that the blood contains too much toxin. This is generally caused by excessive consumption of sugar, cold and synthetic drinks, ice cream and tropical fruit. Anyone with this colouring should go on a strict Ch'ang Ming diet, and thereby cut out the causes.

If the complexion turns dark purple, and shows prominently on the nose, it indicates high blood pressure and an expanded heart. If, in addition, the tongue is also purple coloured, then this is a sign of an enlarged liver and spleen, and internal blood clotting. Counter-measures should be taken as a matter of urgency.

Green. This is a degenerate colour and unfortunately it is becoming more and more common in the Western world, for it is the colour that denotes cancer and it is very Yin indeed. If seen on the left side of the face it is cancer of the liver, and on the right side it is lung cancer.

Glossy. This may also be described as a transparent look or sheen, and sufferers of tuberculosis, leprosy, and some skin complaints, will have this delicate look.

Skin texture, etc.

Roughness. Most Westerners find that when they have become fully mature their skin starts to become rough. This is entirely due to excess consumption of deep-fried foods and meat fats.

Dryness. If the texture of the skin becomes dry, this shows an excessive amount of toxins in the body, affecting the natural oils. This is an instance of contraction, which is Yin.

Perspiration. If, after strenuous physical activity, there is excessive sweating of the face and body, it is generally a sign of over-consumption of fluids. This can cause trouble by over-working the kidneys.

If, however, there has been no physical activity but there is perspiration under the armpits and on the hands, there is trouble in the lungs.

Hair

Colour. White and grey hair on the head is Yin, caused by too much animal meat and dairy products, which have helped to create too much fat in the circulatory system.

Split ends and frizzy hair. Both are Yin and show that there is too much toxin in the body. This is caused especially by over-consumption of fruit, sugar and synthetic drinks. The same symptoms may indicate weaknesses in the sexual organs, i.e. the ovary and testes.

Baldness. This is also Yin. It indicates excessive intake of fluid, fruits and sugar. If these are drastically reduced in your diet this will help to stop your hair from falling out.

Dandruff. This is caused by over-consumption of animal meat and dairy products, and by too great an intake of food generally, which means that you are having too much protein.

Body hair. If an adult person has fine, silvery hair growing on the body this shows an excess of dairy products, and will show up more prominently along the lines of the meridians. If, however, there is excessive hair of normal colour on the body, then look carefully at the position where the hair is growing: if on the chest, then there is trouble in the heart or the lungs; if in the region of the kidneys, then it indicates that the kidneys are over-working.

Face

Shape. The Yin face can be recognised very easily, being long, and coming to a point at the chin, and having a wide forehead. It may be likened to an inverted triangle.

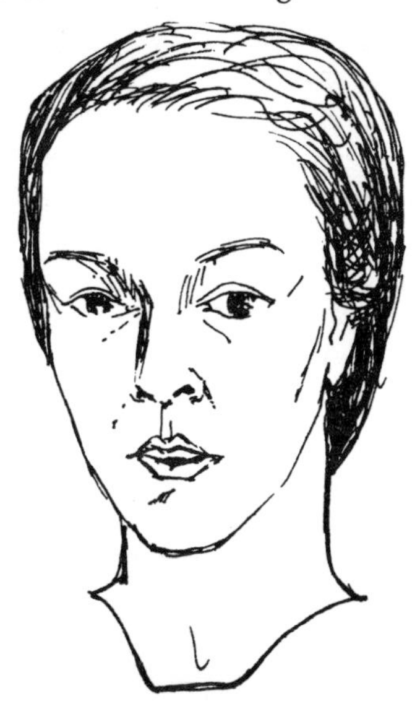

Wrinkles. On a Yin person the wrinkles or lines on the face run vertically. They are caused by the external or macrocosmic energy (Li) returning back to heaven, and because the skin tissue of the person is very weak, it shows up as lines because of the contracting influence.

Vertical lines on the forehead denote a tencency to over-eat, and an over-consumption of meat;

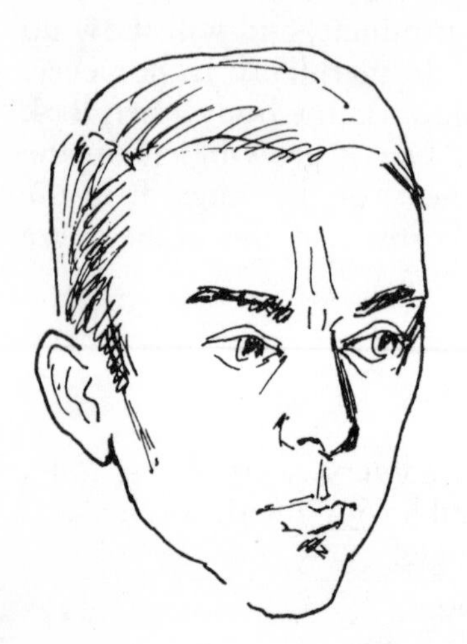

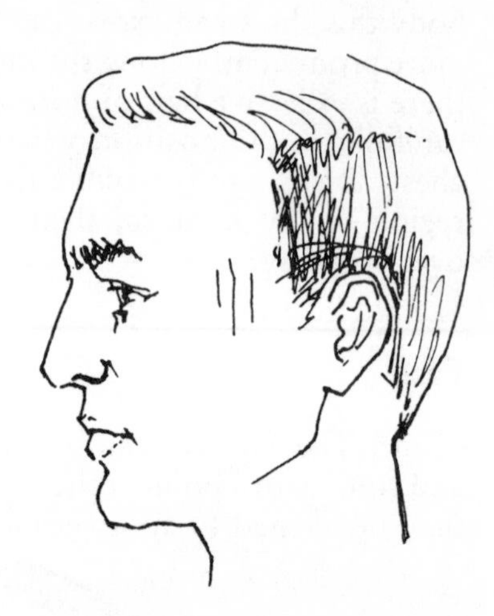

Lines between the eyebrows indicate a bad liver and that the person is very temperamental, so be careful if you are looking for a partner for life, for with a person with such lines you could have a rough time.

Faint, minute vertical lines on the side of the face between the eyes and the ear denote stomach trouble over a very long period.

Pimples. Pimples on the forehead indicate too much shellfish or meat. Pimples on the cheeks mean over-consumption of dairy produce (especially eggs) and chicken. Pimples in the region of the mouth and lower jaw indicate over-eating of meat or salmon. The mere fact that pimples have appeared shows that the system is overloaded and that the body is trying to get rid of the surplus, which it does by this form of discharge.

Black or dark brown pimples are a sign of the discharge of waste products by the body, pimples with white heads generally denote too much toxin in the system or it could mean excessive dairy products or sugar, and red pimples indicate over-consumption of meat or sometimes blood stagnation. So you will appreciate that all pimples tell their own story and indicate specific causes, so it is well worth while to take notice of them.

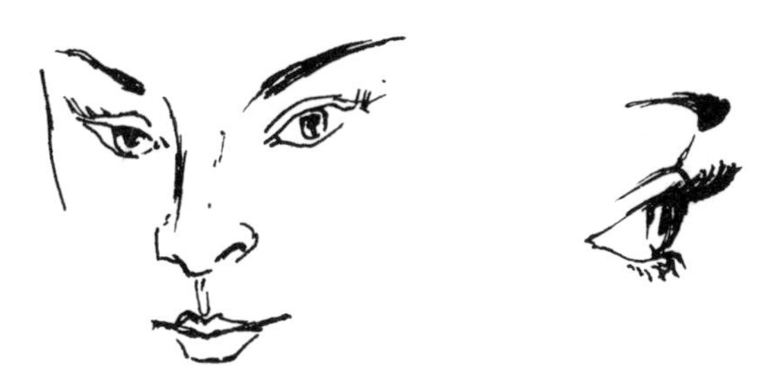

Eyebrows. Thin eyebrows are Yin and are caused by eating too many sweet things, especially sugar. If you keep this up, then you will find your eyebrows will become thinner and thinner until they almost disappear. This can be a dangerous stage for those who have little or no eyebrows are apt to contract cancer.

If the eyebrows turn upwards at the ends, towards the temples, and begin to point above the ears, then you have been eating too much meat for a very long time. It is a sure sign of weakness in the system and also shows a lack of internal energy (Ch'i).

Eyelashes. If they are long that is a Yin sign, and the same is true if they curl upwards. On the other hand, very short or virtually non-existent lashes, which many Western women try to hide by using false eyelashes, is an indication of excessive consumption of animal food. Should a woman who is pregnant have any of these signs, then it indicates that her sexual organs are also Yin, and her baby could also be affected, and so it is vital for her to change to a Ch'ang Ming diet, for the sake of her unborn child.

Eyelids. The eyelids come in two sizes, the double (Yang) and the single (Yin), and the latter is typical of the average Westerner.

Blinking seems to be quite a natural habit that no one pays a lot of attention to it, and least of all, do not appreciate that it can give signs which indicate the health of the body. The less you blink the better is your health, and a truly healthy person should blink only about three to four times per minute. Anyone who blinks less than this is definitely very healthy indeed, and if you hardly blink at all then you are spiritually strong and have very close links with the Tao. If, on the other hand, you blink a lot, then it means that the body is desperately trying to rid itself of the excess Yin influence within the system.

If the eyelid swells up and is continuously swollen, this indicates too great an intake of fluid. If, however, the eyelid remains puffed up after reducing the fluid intake, then there is a possibility of gall-bladder stones.

Eyes

Large Eyes. Large, round eyes are an indication that too much Yin food is being consumed, and that the person concerned is susceptible to colds, influenza and possibly tuberculosis, and in general has very delicate health.

Eyes turned outward. The iris should be in the centre of the eye if healthy, but if the irises are turned outward towards the ears then this is a very Yin sign and indicates excessive toxin in the blood and a danger of cancer.

Following a change to a Ch'ang Ming diet, the irises will eventually re-align themselves to the centre, but the process will be slow.

Low irises. Anyone whose irises lie very low, so that the white of the eye is visible above as well as to the sides of the iris, is a very

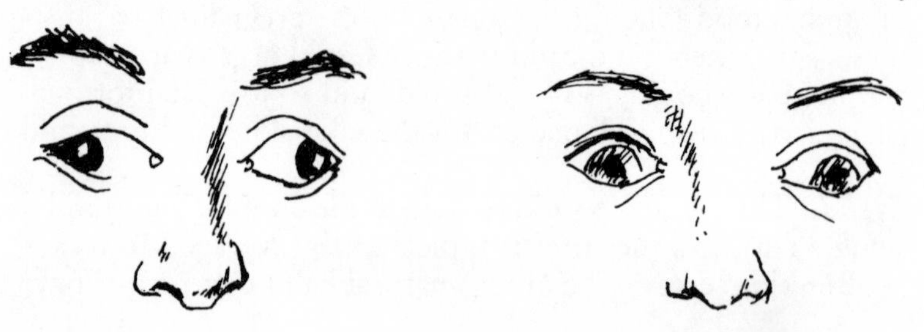

Yin person, showing very deep contraction. Such a person is of unsettled character, having a tendency to argue, abuse and to lose his temper very easily, and is thus prone to be violent and cruel.

Nearsightedness. This occurs when the eyeball has become swollen and enlarged, and it is caused by eating and drinking very Yin foods and drinks over a long period.

Double vision. This is another very Yin symptom and is caused through muscular contraction, which in turn creates tension. Again, this is the result of an excessively Yin diet.

Roving eyes. These are eyes that never stand still, they are on the go continuously first looking one way and then the other, and seem unable to concentrate on anything in particular. This condition is caused by a Yin nervous tension emanating from the heart-governor, and this invariably means a fluctuating heart beat.

Eyeball colours. If the white of the eye is of a yellow colour, then jaundice is indicated; if it is red all over, a bad liver is signified; and a grey or blue colour means that the person is losing his eyesight and may, if these symptoms are ignored, eventually go blind.

If the pupil contracts and the white of the eye turns to a purplish red, then this is a sign of diminished light refraction, reduced vision, with the possibility of colour blindness.

If spots appear on the white of the eyeball close to the iris, certain bodily malfunctions are indicated. Yellow and red spots signify blood stagnation, black indicates kidney problems, green is cancer, and brown denotes the presence of stones or cysts.

Under the eyes. Bags under the eyes will tell their own story. If they happen to look soft and spongy, it is owing to the presence of too much fluid, and shows that the kidneys are being overworked; but, if the swelling under the eyes appears hard in texture, and the complexion is pale, then it is a sure sign of the formation of kidney stones.

A purple or deep blue colouring emanating from the corner of the eye nearest the nose, and creeping down and round the eye, shows that there is blood stagnation. The deeper the colour, the more advanced is the stagnation.

If the edge of the bottom eyelid is white, the person is anaemic, for in a healthy person it will be pink. If it happens to be red, there is inflammation, caused through an infection which has worked its way to the surface, and is an indication of the excessive consumption of sugar, fruit and meat.

Should at any time there be itching inside the bottom eyelid, and with it a feeling as if there is dust or grit in the eye, then take a close look inside the eyelid. If you see minute spots, which are called "granules" there, and have experienced watery eyes and blurred vision, the explanation is Trachoma, and you will appreciate why the Chinese call them "peppery sores" (Chiao Ts'ang). This particular condition is highly infectious, and caused through over-consumption of dairy products, fruit and sugar.

Eye mucus. This is a secretion from the corners of the eye, and if it becomes excessive then the eyelids may become stuck together. This form of discharge should be transparent when the body is healthy, but if it is yellowish then there is an over-consumption of dairy products, and if it is white there is too much toxin in the body, owing to an excess of animal fats. In a woman, excessive eye mucus will also be accompanied by an abnormal, very thick discharge from the vagina. This discharge will have the same discoloration as the mucus.

Nose. A long, thin nose is Yin, and small nostrils denote weak lungs, which is also Yin, and it shows an over-indulgence in Yin foods and drinks, such as ice cream and imitation fruit drinks or it is an excessive intake of drugs and medicaments.

It may surprise you to know that you can see aspects of the heart from the size and condition of the end of the nose. For a bulbous nose shows that the heart has become enlarged and due unfortunately to over-consumption of dairy products, animal meat fats, fruit and alcohol.

A red bulbous nose, means that the blood capillaries are under pressure and are showing through the weak skin tissue. This indicates high blood pressure, and if not corrected it can in time lead to heart trouble or even heart disease. If left too long,

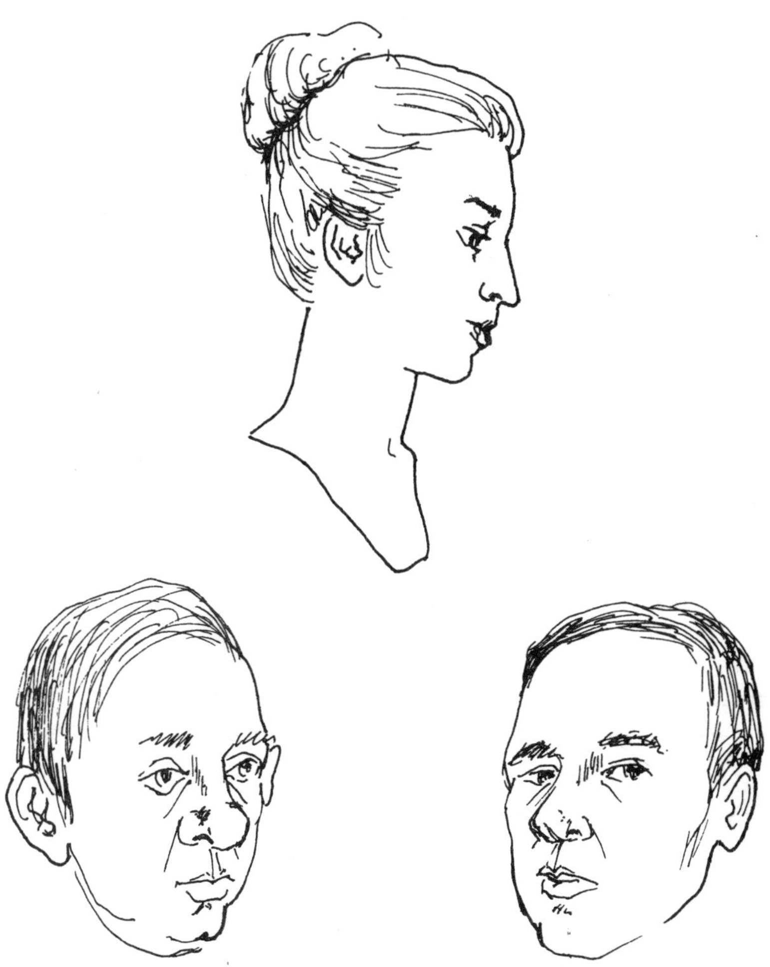

then it can go the other way, to hypotension or low blood pressure, which will then take a long time to cure.

A cleft or vertical line in the middle of the nose denotes that the two chambers of the heart are not working in harmony together, perhaps because one has become enlarged or has shrunk in comparison with the other. The resulting lack of co-ordination produces irregular beating, which is commonly called heart murmur. If you were born of Yin parents then you could have inherited it at birth; or it could have developed simply through bad eating and drinking habits.

If you should suffer from spasmodic nose bleeding, without any apparent reason, this indicates that the tissues of the body are thin and weak, and that either the blood is too thick or there is too much of it. This is caused by an excessive intake of liquids, fruit and fruit juices, sugar or too much protein.

Mouth. When you look at the mouth you are also looking at the condition and state of the person's stomach and intestines. For instance, a big mouth will show that there is a swelling within the stomach and thereby denotes a degeneration of the digestive system, especially the intestines.

Lips. If the lips are thin this shows a Yin person, and if one lip is larger than the other this also is Yin, for both lips should be of the same thickness. If a person with thin lips also has a tendency to pucker them constantly, then it indicates deep contractive influence and is very Yin indeed. If the upper lip is swollen then there is a weakness in the stomach, and if the bottom lip is swollen then the intestines are in trouble.

Dry lips indicate that there is too much toxin in the body, and this is very common in the West, which is why many women use a lot of cream. If the lips become chapped, then there is definitely some internal upsets, in the stomach (upper lip) or in the intestines (lower lip). If cracks should appear on the lips, then do something about it fast, for the trouble is becoming acute. The position of the crack will tell you the organ that is affected.

In a healthy person the lips are pink. Darker lips which are becoming very common indicate over-consumption of Yin foods, including meat, and people with dark lips tend to have the more serious illnesses, including cancer. Dark red lips on a person who also has a red face is a sure sign of excess heat in the lungs which in turn can indicate fever, internal inflammation, constipation, and headaches. People with very pale lips tend to be anaemic, and pale lips are also a sign of scarlet fever.

A cyst on the lips indicates a cyst, ulcer or tumour in the stomach (upper lip), intestines (lower lip), or the duodenum (corner of the mouth). The trouble should, however, be evident before the cysts actually appear, and counter-measures should be taken as soon as possible.

Teeth. If the body is truly healthy then all the teeth should be of a normal size and uniform in shape, and you will never get cavities in them. Protruding teeth are Yin, and so are teeth with gaps between them. In fact, in China it is understood that protruding teeth indicate a person who will always want to be on the go, and that people with gaps between the teeth will separate from their parents, and also from their spouses, at some time or another.

There are only two ways you can get bad, weak or pointed teeth (all very Yin signs); and these are through bad blood or bad saliva. If the blood is bad, then there is an over-consumption of meat and meat products, sugar and fruit, or too many drugs and medicines are being taken. Or it is the saliva that is at fault, the cause may be vinegar or synthetic drinks.

Gums. Healthy gums are pink, if they happen to be red then there is blood stagnation, and if white then there is anaemia. If they are yellow, there are many possible causes and reasons, the most likely being severe jaundice.

If the gums are soft and spongy, this shows that too much liquid has been consumed over a long period, and that there is too much toxin in the body; so reduce your fluid intake, and cut out animal fats, sugar, fruit and synthetic drinks.

The Tongue. This book is not big enough to explain every single illness and disease of which the tongue can tell us, especially when you appreciate that it has a reciprocal relationship to the four major organs of the body, and its condition is thus extremely important in the art of diagnosis. In China this is how we relate the tongue to the organs:

The tip of the tongue is the eye of the heart.
The two sides of the tongue are the eyes of the liver.
The root of the tongue is the eye of the kidneys.
The middle of the tongue is the eye of the stomach.

Look into the eyes of the tongue and you will see all, and through the medium of the other diagnostic observations you will be able to obtain definite confirmation of the illnesses and diseases that are predominant in the body.

If the tongue is red then there is heart trouble, and the same is indicated where a crack or furrow runs from the tip of the tongue down its centre. If the mouth, throat and lips are dry, with the tip of the tongue coloured red, then the lungs are in trouble, with the possibility of bronchitis.

If the sides of the tongue are red, liver trouble is indicated, and redness of the root or middle of the tongue indicates trouble in the kidneys or stomach, respectively. If the tongue becomes smooth and shiny, this is further confirmation.

If the tongue trembles when the mouth is open, then it shows that the nervous system is under stress, or it could mean that there is trouble within the brain.

Should the tongue be purple in colour, it is a sign of blood stagnation and therefore the liver and possibly the spleen are enlarged. This means that there is a danger of liver abscesses and hepatitis.

If there is yellow furring of the tongue, there is something radically wrong, for yellow indicates excess toxin and acidity in the system.

Should any areas of the tongue appear black, this could mean that there is a possibility of cancer.

Sputum. This is another major aid to diagnosis, for almost every conceivable complaint will show up in the sputum or the lack of it, in its colours, smoothness, foaminess and so on. The following are a few examples.

Bronchial asthma	–	White foamy sputum.
Tuberculosis	–	Thick yellow sputum.
Whooping cough	–	White smooth sputum.
Lobar pneumonia	–	Rusty coloured sputum.
Tonsilitis	–	White sputum.
Lung abscess	–	Purulent sputum.
Cardiac disease	–	Pink sputum.

Any coloration of the sputum is an indicator of ill health, for it should be colourless and there should be very little of it. Excessive liquid intake tends to increase the amount of sputum.

Ears. The ears indicate the balance within the circulation of the body and the state of the kidneys. For instance, high pointed ears, or ears that stick out, and small ears which limit the area of receptive sound, and ears without lobes are all signs of Yin influence and excess consumption of animal meat and fats. This contractive influence will also show up in the character and personal emotions.

A red ear will show that there is kidney infection, blood stagnation, or both, owing to excessive consumption of meat and salt, which produces acidity.

Ear troubles are on the increase and so are the numbers of those who become totally deaf, mainly due to faulty eating and drinking habits, but how good is your own hearing? To test the condition of your ears, put a finger into each ear in turn, and see, when you withdraw it, if the tip of the finger is wet. If it is, then your hearing is already impaired and has become faulty, and you have lost about twenty to thirty per cent of your hearing ability, through consumption of too much meat, dairy products, sugar and fruit.

If, however, the fluid in your ear starts to solidify into a thick glutinous substance, this is a sign of real trouble, which cleaning the ear cannot eradicate, for it will occur time and time again if steps are not taken to prevent it. Then there will come a time when you are totally deaf, through solidification of the mucus, which stops the three bones of the auditory ossicles from moving and thereby the auditory nerve can no longer oscillate. To prevent this, avoid the foods mentioned above, and cut out ice cream, drugs and medicines.

Hands. Put your hand flat on the table and raise the fingers. There should be at least a two-inch gap between the tips of the fingers and the table. Now, keeping the palm flat on the table, lift the fingers with the other hand. There should be a three or four-inch gap between the tips of your fingers and the table. Finally, keeping your hand on the table, lift your elbow so that your whole forearm is perpendicular, i.e. at right angles to the hand. In all three tests, you should feel no pain or stress whatsoever, and if, because of stiffness in the finger joints or the wrist you cannot fulfil them, this is a sure sign of hardening of the arteries, owing to too much cholesterol. Most people will expect the old to have this stiffness, which is a Yin symptom, but that is

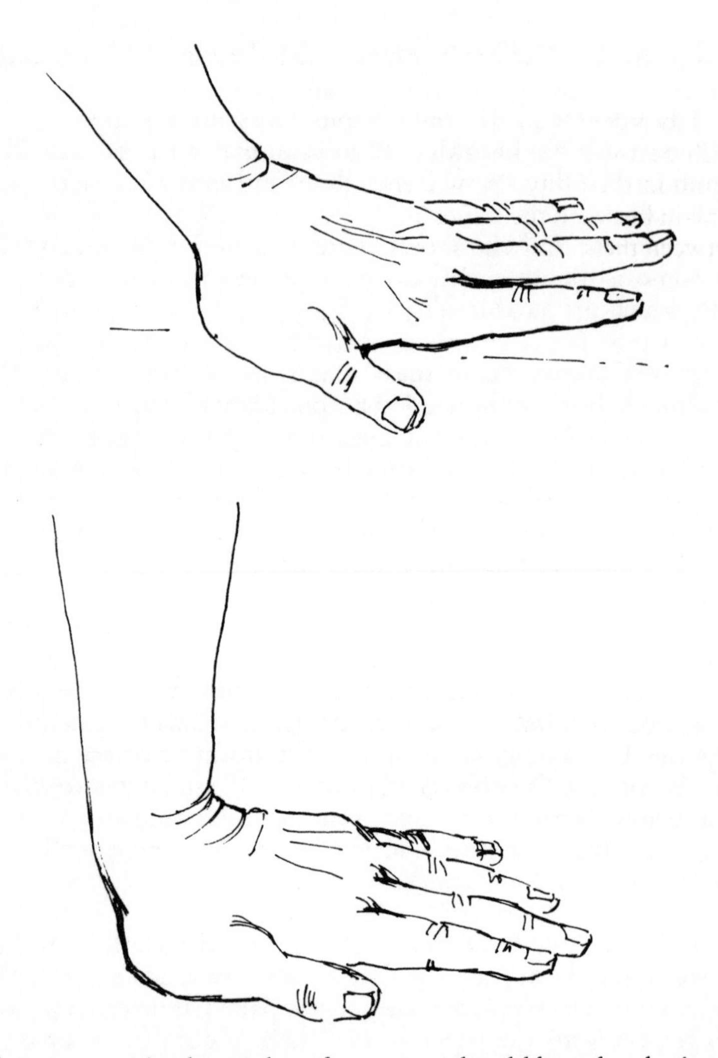

the wrong attitude to adopt for no one should have hardening of the arteries, not even the very, very old, for the arteries are the life line of the body. Cholesterol is created by consuming meat or meat fats, dairy products, various nut butters and deep-fried foods.

A narrow palm and long, thin, delicate-looking fingers are Yin signs, indicative of a weak and sensitive health, and if care is not taken a person with such symptoms could catch almost any illness or disease in their lifetime, including nervous and emotional upsets.

Lay your hand flat on the table. Do you have loose flabby flesh between the knuckles? If you do, then there is too much liquid in the body. Now clench that hand into a fist, and again look in between the knuckles. If there is no valley or indentation between them, this also shows a hardening of the arteries, and too an excess of fluid, so that the kidneys are swollen.

Clench one hand into a fist, then rub the back of it with the other hand. If it feels dry to the touch, this is a Yin sign and indicates that there is too much toxin in the body. If you pull the skin on the back of the hand, it should spring back immediately you let it go; if not, and it feels thick and stiff, again there is too much toxin in the body, through over-consumption of animal fats, sugar and fruit.

Now have a look at the veins on the back of the hand. If they bulge out, there is too much fluid in the body. Whilst you are looking at the back of your hand, see if the fingers are trembling. If they are, then this is an outward sign of a nervous complaint, and it is related to the heart governor.

The colour of the palm is a very good indication of the health of the body. White or pale hands indicate anaemia, deep red signifies blood stagnation or that the body has undergone a change of diet. Yellow palms can signify jaundice, with the spleen and pancreas as the main sources of the trouble, but it can also show that a malfunction of the gall bladder or that there could also be a liver infection. Purple or blue palms show that there is an over-consumption of sweets, sugar, and fruits.

If the palms feel hot and wet, this points to liver trouble, but, if they are cold and damp, lung troubles are indicated. If the hands feel just warm but wet, there is too much fluid in the system.

Nails. No matter how much nail varnish is used you cannot hide the bad health of the body, only disguise the colour of the nails. There are many tell-tale signs that can easily be seen, and which tells the world how Yin that person really is. For instance, long and narrow nails are Yin and so are nails that are flat, when viewed from the front. Concave nails which are sometimes referred to as hollow or spoon-shaped, are a sign of worms present in

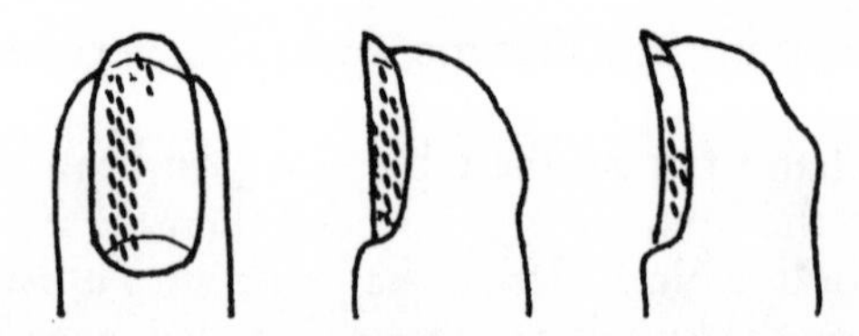

the body, and which have been there for some considerable time; and so are cracked nails too, and all due to animal meat or in some cases, to unwashed vegetables, but mainly the former. If some-one continuously bites their nails, have a look at them when the opportunity permits, and if they are cracked or concave, or both, then they certainly have had worms over a very long period of time.

If there are half moons at the bottom of the nails, then this is another sign of Yin, for it shows that there is too much toxin in the body. The bigger the moons, the greater amount of toxin. If there is truly good health then you will find that there are no moons at all on the fingers, and only a very small half moon on the thumb.

Pink nails are a sign of good health, whilst deep red nails shows that the blood has an excess of protein, owing to too much meat, whilst white nails indicate that the person is anaemic, and yellow nails are a sign of jaundice, and malfunctioning of the spleen, pancreas and liver.

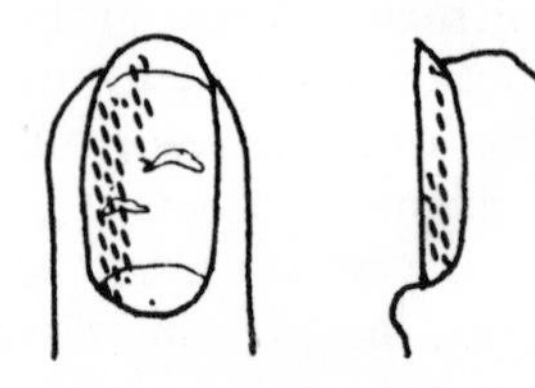

If there are any white spots on the nails, a strong sugar, chemical or drug intake in indicated, and as it takes nine to ten months for the nail to grow from bottom to top, the position of the spot is a clear indicator of when the excess was consumed. For instance, if you have a good time at Christmas, then watch out for the spots, for they will be over halfway up the nail by June.

Now have a look at the flesh at the base of the nails. If it is thick and raised, and very red and has a tendency to peel, or has been nibbled away, there is excess protein in the body, owing to over-consumption of meat products. The person is also likely to be very nervous.

Height. A tall person is Yin, and more and more Westerners are becoming very tall, owing to excess consumption of very Yin foods, by themselves and by their parents before them. Very thin, skinny people are also Yin. The ideal height is seven times that of the size of the head measured from the chin to the crown.

Walking. Bow legs are Yin, and it shows that mother over-fed her baby and that there was too much animal meat and salt included in the diet. Pigeon toes, or walking with the toes turned in, is also Yin, for it is a sign of contraction. So are rounded shoulders or a stooping posture. It is also Yin to walk with the weight of the body on the toes, a fact of which high-heel shoes take advantage.

For the hips to swing from side to side is very Yin, and it is another Western idea of beauty and sex appeal, and if a girl stands with both feet together, and there is a gap between the upper thighs, this is also Yin, and is a sign that the person is very emotional.

Weight. It is Yin to be underweight, and to get an approximate idea of the correct weight that you should be, here is a simple way to work it out. First of all multiply every inch over five feet by five, and then add 110. The result is the number of pounds that you should weigh. So, if you are five feet six inches tall, you should weigh 140 lb, or ten stone (6 inches × 5 = 30 + 110 = 140). For a man, add a further seven pounds to obtain the absolute maximum weight; and, for a woman, deduct seven pounds to ascertain the minimum weight limit that you should be. So, for someone five feet six inches tall, it would work out like this:

	Minimum weight	Maximum weight
Man	140 lb	147 lb
Woman	133 lb	140 lb

Abdomen. Normally no one takes any notice of their abdomen until it starts to ache or swell up, at which stage it becomes impossible to ignore.

Pain is something that can only be felt and not seen, so the distension of the abdomen must have an important reason, and whilst there can be many explanations, it is likely to result from an infection or disease of the liver, kidney or heart. Owing to severe and deep contraction, which is very Yin, the excess fluid that has been consumed or created cannot get away, and so the abdomen swells. Among the illnesses that can cause this are cirrhosis of the liver, hepatitis, stomach cancer, stomach ulcers and heart failure.

Bladder. If the bladder swells up, it is usually because of severe contraction, the urine cannot be passed away. This "urine retention" is very Yin, as are bladder stones, which invariably cause inflammation of the bladder which in turn also causes the bladder to swell. Contrary to popular belief, there are no drugs or medicaments that can dissolve these stones, and it may be necessary to have an operation. So the best advice is to eat and drink the Ch'ang Ming way, so that you will not have a tendency to develop them.

Urine. The health of the body can be seen from the urine, and whilst you may not normally see another person's urine, at least they may be able to convey to you their own observations, and you can watch the colour of your own urine, which is secreted through the kidneys and then passed on to the bladder.

Too much liquid will make the kidneys swell, which impairs their efficiency. Normally a person should only consume about one pint of fluid a day, and a good guideline to see if too much fluid is being drunk is that a man should urinate only two or three times daily, and a woman whose bladder is bigger, only once or twice.

Many illnesses and infections affect the colour of the urine and the frequency of urination. Here are a few guidelines to be used in conjunction with other diagnostic observations.

Urine infection – frequent urination.
Epilepsy – loses control of urine emission.

Tuberculosis	urine a dark yellow, and urinates frequently.
Gastro-enteritis –	not much urine passed, and it will be yellow.
Liver cirrhosis	scant amount of urine and yellow coloured.
Leukaemia	sometimes a little blood in the urine.
Dysentery	urine brown, and only a little of it.
Hepatitis	urine a dark reddish yellow and appears foamy.

The lighter coloured the urine, the more Yin the influence, so it is advisable to cut down on the quantity of liquid consumed, and also cut out all fruits and sugar.

Stools. Everyone should get into the habit of passing their motion at least once every day, and it is a very good habit to do so at the same time each day. The best time is when you get up in the morning, so that you can rid yourself of all the waste built up the previous day and start the new day afresh.

In the case of a normal, healthy person the stools or faeces will be brown and firm. If they tend to be watery, there is over-consumption of fluid, fruit and sugar. If they happen to be very dark or appear black, then too much animal meat is being consumed.

There should be no smell, but, if they do smell putrid, it is a sign of infection in the stomach or the large intestine. Black, tarry coloured stools with streaks of blood could indicate stomach cancer, ulcers or cirrhosis of the liver, but, if there are streaks of blood in a motion of normal colour, it may indicate bleeding in the rectum, leukaemia, dysentery, intestinal infection, or, in some cases, anaemia.

If the motion is small or you get constipation, it is a sign of Yin contraction, and you should give your bowels a rest by not eating so much and by making sure that you chew your food really well. If, however, the stool breaks away into fragments, this could mean worms, so watch all the symptoms carefully.

Are you Yang?

Skin colour. If you are truly healthy, your skin should be a glowing pink, and throughout the year, summer or winter, it should be constantly warm to the touch with no variation whatsoever.

A red complexion of an adult shows that he or she is Yang, but has a tendency to be too Yang, caused either through too much protein, excess consumption of meat or to having too much blood in the system. If the skin colour changes with the heat of the summer or cold in the winter, then these are Yin changes and indicates ill health.

Red skin in a very young baby is quite normal for as it grows and expands it slowly becomes more Yang, and therefore will be glowing with the vitality and energy that is typical of its growth.

Skin texture. The skin should be smooth to the touch, just like feeling velvet, with enough oil in the tissue to keep it flexible, and it is this oil in the skin that helps to give a glow to the complexion.

Artificial oils and cream do not replace the natural oils of the body, but, in fact they have a tendency to block the pores, thereby making the body unhygienic and preventing the tissues from breathing properly. This lack of air in the tissue allows cancer to rear its ugly head and to spread very fast.

Hair. Black hair is Yang, red hair is even more Yang, and ginger hair is very Yang. The hair should be shiny in its natural state, that is without anything being put on to it.

Naturally wavy or curly hair is also Yang, and the hair should be strong, and if you wish to know if your hair is truly healthy, just take a strand of it from your head, and see if you can break it. If your hair is healthy it will not break.

If the hair is dry then it has become too Yang, and you need a little more oil in the diet. This can be obtained by sautéing your vegetables regularly, and by eating them with a little seaweed that has been boiled for a long time and to which tea oil (or, if you cannot obtain that, sesame oil) and soya sauce have been added. Depending on the type of seaweed that you can get, you will need to boil it three to five hours to get the maximum benefit from it.

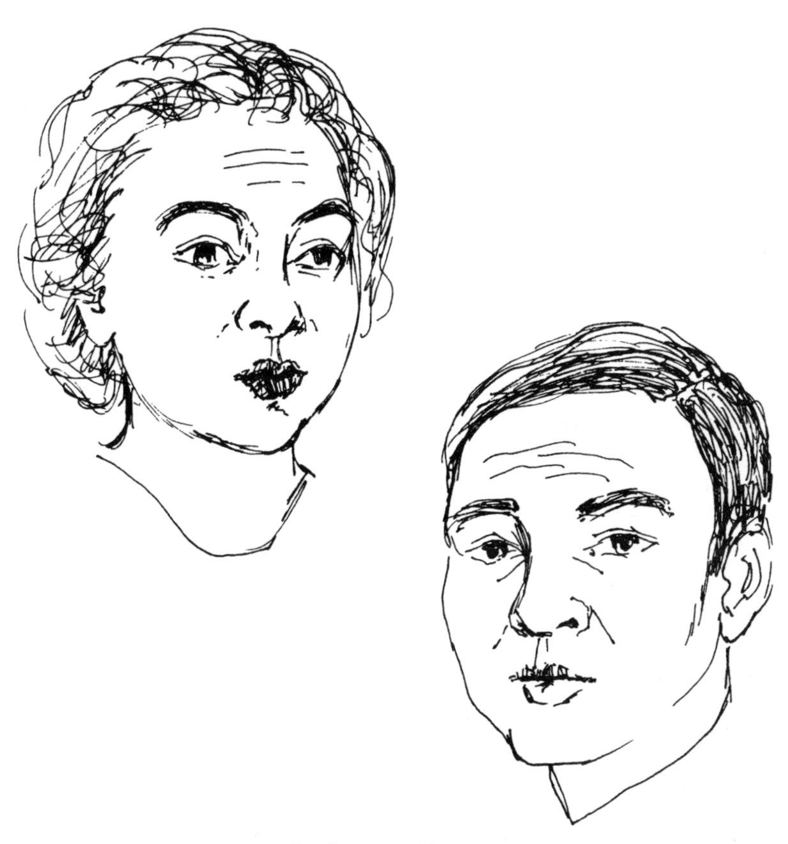

Face. In a Yang person the face and head should be round and the chin square. Horizontal lines running across the forehead, providing they are parallel to one another, indicate that the person has an orderly mind, is an extremely good organiser, and has a well advanced brain.

If, however, these lines tend to waver a lot, look a bit erratic, or go off in different directions, the person is apt to be chaotic in his thinking, even to the point of being schizophrenic.

In a truly Yang person, there will be no lines in between the eyebrows, and, even if you pucker your eyebrows, you will not be able to make any lines appear.

Eyebrows. A thick and broad eyebrow is Yang, and it should follow the natural curvature of the eye.

Eyelashes. The eyelashes should be strong and straight, and should not curl at all. Those that do curl up are Yin, for they are leaving the eyeball unprotected. Whilst the surface of the eye is kept clean by the secretions of the lacrimal glands, the first line of defence of the eyes is the eyelashes, which need to be straight if they are to perform their function correctly.

Eyelids. In countries that have a lot of glaring sunshine, it is normal for people to have double eyelids. This is for protection and is Yang.

Eyes. Long thin eyes are Yang, and the iris when settled should be exactly in the centre of the eye, so that all the retinal cells receive an equal quantity of light.

Cross eyes show that the person has become too Yang, and that there is far too much toxin within the system, and therefore there is a tendency towards high blood pressure. People with cross eyes should start on a Ch'ang Ming diet as soon as they can, for it will help the eyes to change back to normal. This, however, is a long, slow process, so don't expect a change to happen over-night.

Nose. A short nose is Yang, and if it is slightly turned up at the end, then this is an even stronger Yang sign. It is also Yang if the nose is broad and the nostrils large.

Mouth. A mouth that is small is very Yang, for the average size of a Yang mouth, from corner to corner is equal to the width of the nose.

Lips. Pink lips are Yang, for they show that the body is healthy. Thick lips are also Yang, providing that both lips are the same size. However, do not mistake swollen lips as thick lips, for swollen lips are very Yin and may denote epilepsy.

Teeth. Teeth that are evenly distributed and of normal size and shape create a balance to the mouth, and this is Yang. There should be no gaps at all, and the teeth should be upright. If, however, the teeth slopc inward, this is a sign of being too Yang.

Gums. In a truly healthy person the gums should be pink and firm, and if this is their condition then it is Yang.

Tongue. A pink tongue is a sign of good health and therefore denotes a Yang condition, and the surface should be like the skin of a strawberry, with little undulations and a very slight roughness.

Ears. Good Yang signs are big ears and big lobes, and ears that lie against the head. Anything else is Yin.

Hands. A thick, round, pink palm, and short, stocky fingers are Yang and thereby signify good health. The hands should always be warm and no matter what the weather conditions might be, they should always be dry.

Nails. It is Yang and a sign of good health when the grain of the nails run from bottom to top, and so are:

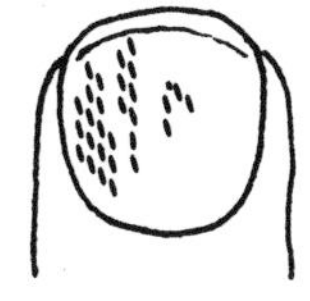

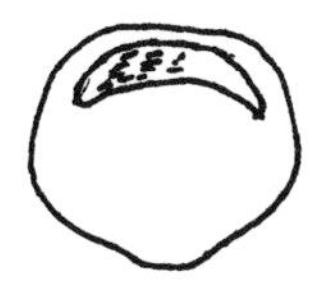

short and wide nails and so are rounded nails

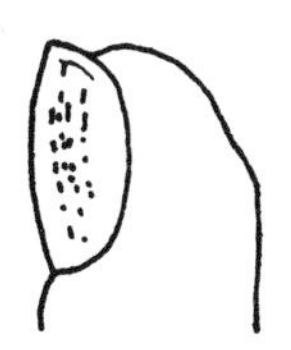

and nails that are convex in shape.

There should be no half moons at the bottom of the nails, except, perhaps, for a very small one on the thumbnails. The nails should be very hard without being brittle, and they should be pink. Watch them carefully, for they are the windows of your blood.

Height. Being short and stocky is Yang, but this depends on the size of the head in relation to the overall height as outlined earlier.

Walking. A woman with a Yang hip swing walks so that her dress or slacks creases diagonally from the buttock to the hip, which also means that she will be stockily built in her old age.

If the hip rolls up and down on the outside, then the person is overweight for her build and needs to go on a Ch'ang Ming diet. Otherwise, as she grows older she will suffer increasing stresses, and in her middle age she will be very fat.

Urine. If you are eating the Ch'ang Ming way daily then your urine should be the colour of China tea, a medium tone of yellow, neither too dark not too light, and there should be no smell to it.

Stools. If you are Yang your motion should be brown, firm and long, but this can be affected by changes in the diet, such as having too much salt, or consuming extra dairy products.

It is natural that you will first take a look at yourself to see which category you come under, and then having fully assessed every point that has been mentioned, no doubt you will want to start eating and drinking the Ch'ang Ming way so that you can attain permanent good health. You will then fully appreciate, in time, what the Yin and Yang really means, and how you can create the balance of the two within yourself.

Chapter 7

Symptoms of Illness

In the previous chapter we examined the outward signs of the body's health, as indicated by their various Yin and Yang characteristics. In this chapter we group these symptoms under specific illnesses and weaknesses (and we list them alphabetically, for easy reference), adding a number of general symptoms where necessary, especially those that convey no outward signs of their existence.

Naturally, we hope that by doing it this way you will have a greater understanding and appreciation of the illnesses that humanity suffers, and how the body shows its objection and its efforts in trying to reject each one.

In Chinese traditional therapy there are eight classifications of diseases all of which can be simply divided into Yin and Yang categories.

Yin Illnesses: Internal (nei), cold (han) and deficient (hsu). The general symptoms of these are pale, transparent complexion, weariness, shallow breathing, poor appetite, cold hands and feet, damp hands and dampness under armpits, a pale tongue with a white furring, urinates frequently although fluid intake is generally low, has a tendency to drink warm or hot drinks, motions are loose, quiet in attitude and speech, likes to keep to himself avoiding crowds whenever possible, and has a sunken, slow, deficient or weak pulse.

Yang Illnesses: External (wai), hot (je) and solid (ying). The general outlines of a person with a Yang illness are, a flushed complexion, a very warm body so is always looking for the coolest spot, loud mouthed and very talkative, and likes company, always restless, rough and loud breathing, always thirsty so consumes a lot of fluid, dry mouth and generally has cracked lips, a deep red or purplish coloured tongue with yellow furring, has a burning sensation when passing urine which is only in small amounts, constipated, and has a floating, rapid, tight or forceful pulse.

However, the Yin and Yang complaints and symptoms do overlap each other and can therefore make diagnosis a little complex, especially as not all the symptoms may appear at the same time or in any one person, but experience will help to overcome any deficiency in the manifestation of an illness.

Naturally, the number of ailments covered here must be limited, but we will deal with the most basic and common ones that exist, and ones that you will no doubt come across fairly frequently in your lifetime.

Acidosis of the blood.
Cross eyes
Enlarged pupils

Anaemia.
White complexion
White hair
White nails
Edge of the bottom eyelid white
Smooth, shiny tongue
Cracks at the corners of the mouth
White or pale coloured hands
Lassitude
Swollen ankles
Breathlessness
Dyspepsia
Spots before the eyes
Dizziness
Diarrhoea
Easily fatigued

Animal meat—over-consumption of.
Long eyelashes
Redness in the white of the eye
Eyebrows that curve up at the outer end
Loss of hair on the crown of the head
Vertical lines on the forehead
Fat bulbous nose, that is sometimes shiny
Dark lips
Red ears
Pointed teeth
Red complexion

Swollen and thick cuticles
Red and peeling skin on the cuticles
Has a tendency to pick or nibble the cuticles
Very big half-moons on the nails
Skin on the back of the hand does not retract quickly
Red nails
Bow legs
Putrid smell to the breath

Anus trouble.
Persistent rectal irritation
The heel of the palm dark red
Pain when passing motion
Sometimes a hard swelling is felt
Motion may be streaked with blood

Blood alkalosis.
Blood too alkaline
Both eyes turned outward
Apprehension, anxiety and worry are predominant

Blood circulation poor.
Dark lips
Face and especially the nose turns red in the cold weather

Blood pressure high.
Cross eyes
Red capillaries at the tip of the nose
Dizziness
Tiredness
Pain in the chest
Ringing in the ears
Occasionally there may be misty vision

Blood stagnation.
Swelling under the eyes
Purple or dark blue colouring under the eyes
Dark lips
Black or dark-purple gums
Face and especially the nose turns red in cold weather

Red ears
Red hands
Skin ulcers
Stomach ache
Purple tongue
Sometimes headaches occur

Bladder trouble.
Heel of the palm dark red
Fatigue
Urination is frequent and painful
Loss of weight
Dryness in the throat
Yellow fur on the tongue
Cloudy urine
Poor appetite
Sometimes accompanied by chills or fever
Aches in knees and back
Moodiness
Pink tongue
Bitter taste in the mouth

Bones weak.
Tooth decay
Weak teeth
Anaemia

Brain troubles.
Tongue cannot be stretched out straight
Tongue trembles
Eyes constantly on the move
Trembling fingers and hands
Irritation
Hallucinations may occur

Bronchial asthma.
Foamy white sputum
Sometimes sputum is grey and it may be streaked with blood
Lips and face red
Wheezing

Dislikes cold weather
Dry stools
Yellow urine
Anxiety
Body sometimes gets hot
Breathlessness
Inability to sleep, restlessness, night sweats
Loss of weight
Dry mouth
Sometimes chills or fever

Cancer.
Both eyes turned outward
Green complexion
Almost no eyebrows
Dark lips
Jaundice
Anaemia
Frequent headaches
Chest pains
Weight loss
Root of the tongue black
Swollen abdomen
Loss of appetite
Nausea
Tarry stools

Cardiac disease.
Purplish lips
Pink sputum
Palpitations
Rapid heart-beat
Coughing

Chemicals and drugs, over-consumption.
White spots will appear on the nails

Cholestrol, too much.
Fingers cannot be bent back
Wrist cannot be bent back to a 90-degree angle

Colds.

Physical condition is generally poor
Furred tongue
Big eyes
Throat painful
White or very pale complexion
Tongue may be coloured yellow, white or red

Constipation.

Lower lip swollen
Furred tongue, which may be coloured white, yellow or purple
Sometimes putrid wind
Depression
Spasms of the colon
Chemicals irritating the intestine
Face flushed
Swollen abdomen
Sometimes lips very pale or black
Stools hard, dry and thick

Cruel personality.

Irises at the bottom of the eye

Diabetes.

One iris looks towards the nose; the other is normal
Itching around the urinary outlet
Septic spots
Ulcers on the feet
Feet and shins become painful
Cramp
Nerve pains in the limbs
Constipation
Sometimes boils recurring
Sore, red, dry throat, and gets thirsty often
Tongue furred yellow
Dry skin
Blurred vision

Dysentry.

Urine brown, and only small amounts are passed at any one time
Sometimes face and lips turn a bluish green
Blood in the motion
Nausea
Vomiting
Headaches
Painful abdomen
Intestine noises
Eyes red
Stools change colour
Sometimes feverish

Epilepsy.

Both lips swollen
Complexion blank and pale
Spasms at the corners of the mouth
Dilated pupils
Sometimes the white of the eye can be seen above or below the iris
A loud cry emitted at beginning of an attack
Sometimes becomes unconscious
Foaming at the mouth
Body convulsions

Female sexual organs, trouble with.

Dark brown colour under the eyes
A horizontal line between the upper lip and nose
Dark lips and dark gums show irregular periods
Split ends and frizzy hair

Gall-bladder stones.

Swelling around the eyes, particularly the upper eyelid
A yellow tint in the white of the eye
Nausea
White or yellowish fur on the tongue

Gall-bladder trouble.

Symptoms are similar to gall-bladder stones

Yellow complexion
Palms of the hands yellowish

Gastro-enteritis.
Urine yellow and very little of it
Gassy and foul-smelling motions
Chills and fever occur
Watery stools
Abdominal pains
Bad eating habits

Heart abnormal.
Pupils of the eyes too big
Red complexion
Red, bulbous nose
Generally a weak constitution

Heart-governor trouble.
Eyes constantly on the move
Eyes react sluggishly
Trembling fingers and hands

Heart murmur.
Cleft in the middle of the nose

Heart trouble.
Enlarged and bulbous nose
Red-tipped nose
Red tongue that is smooth and shiny
Purplish lips
Deep crack down the middle of the tongue
Red face
Swollen abdomen

Hepatitis.
Foamy dark reddish-yellow urine
Pink tongue
Yellow fur on the tongue
Sometimes the abdomen may be distended
Bitter taste in the mouth
Nausea

Vomiting
Poor appetite
Aversion to greasy foods
Sometimes chills or fever
Restlessness
Thirsty
Headaches

Intestine trouble.
Pimples on the face
Swollen lower lip
Red rash may appear
Side of the thumb turns blue
White or yellow fur on the tongue
Nausea
Abdominal pains that feel like cramps
Vomiting
Scanty urination
Thirsty
May break out in sweats

Jaundice.
Yellow gums
Palms of the hands turn yellow
Abdominal distention
Poor appetite
Nausea
Vomiting
Body and face may turn a yellow colour
Extremities of the arms and legs may feel cold
A feeling of weakness
Whites of the eyes turn yellow
White or yellow fur on the tongue
Sometimes feel dizzy after having a meal
Small stools in the motion

Kidney trouble.
Dark brown colour under the eyes
Red ears
Black or dark brown complexion

Swollen abdomen
Swelling under the eyes
Tiredness
Back aches
Poor appetite
Nausea
Watery stools
Headaches

Leukemia.
Sometimes blood in the urine and in the motion
Anaemia
Tendency to bleed
High fever over a long period
Pale complexion
Headaches
Aches and pains in the body
Dizziness
Weight loss
Swollen abdomen
Diarrhoea

Liver trouble.
Apt to be emotional
Whites of the eye become reddish
Vertical lines between the eyes
Yellow complexion
Yellow palms and fingers
Blue or white complexion (if patient drinks alcohol)
Blue blood capillaries, especially on the temples
Dandruff
Red sides of the tongue
Sometimes the tongue may change to a purple colour
Swollen upper lip
Yellow nails
Swollen abdomen
Yellow urine and only a little of it
Tenderness in the liver area
Poor appetite
Swelling in the legs

Lobar pneumonia.

Rust coloured sputum
Shivering
Vomiting
Pain on one side of the chest
Reddish complexion tinged with blue
Thin furring on the tongue
Lips dry
Sometimes delirious at night

Lung trouble.

Small nostrils
White skin like porcelain
Purulent sputum which may sometimes be either yellow or green
Poor appetite
Coughing
Sometimes a dull pain in the chest
Sometimes feverish
White or pale yellow furring on the tongue

Male sexual organs, trouble with.

Horizontal line between the upper lip and the nose
Dark lips
Split ends and frizzy hair

Menstruation troubles.

Dark gums
Dark lips
Tip of the tongue red
Purple or blue colour under the eyes
Dry skin
Menses dark red or purple
Cold hands and feet
Dizziness
Lack of energy
Clots in the menstruation
Yellow urine
Yellow fur on the tongue
Backache

Painful abdomen
Weakness in the legs and loins
Loss of appetite
Bad-tempered

Nervous-system trouble.
Tongue cannot be stretched out straight
Tongue trembles
Fingers tremble
Eyes constantly on the move
Red and peeling cuticles
Chewing of nails or cuticles
Dizziness
Headaches
Cannot concentrate
Bad tempered
Insomnia
Sometimes spots before the eyes
Fatigue

Nose bleeding.
Weak body tissue
Blood too thick
Too much blood
High blood pressure

Protein, over-consumption of.
Pimples or sties on the interior of the eyelid
Dandruff
Symptoms also listed under "Animal meat, over-consumption of"

Salt, too much.
Bow legs
Red ears
Dry skin
Weak heart
Constipation
High blood pressure
Fatigue

Insomnia
Dark skin
Protruding teeth
Rusty-coloured urine

Scarlet fever.
Pale lips
Sore red throat
Pimply tongue
Skin peels in big patches
Abdominal pains
Fever
Flushed cheeks
Vomiting
Furred tongue

Schizophrenia.
Erratic horizontal lines across the forehead
Bizarre emotions
Physical weakness
Diminished internal energy and diverted external energy

Sinusitis.
Stopped up nose
Loss of smell
Headaches
Dizziness
Feeling of heaviness in the head
Concentration falters
Poor appetite
Sticky and purulent nasal discharge
Occasional fever
Poor memory

Skin changes.
Chapped lips
Dandruff
Flaking skin

Spleen and pancreas trouble.

Yellow face
Yellow palms
Yellow fingers
Yellow nails
Purple tongue

Stomach trouble.

Redness in the middle of the tongue
Redness also showing at the root of the tongue
Cysts at the right or left sides of the mouth
Chapped lips
White tongue
Yellow complexion
Side of the thumb shows a bluish tint

Stomach ulcers.

Symptoms are similar to stomach trouble
Swollen abdomen
Tarry stools
Stomach pains, especially after meals
Sometimes the motion may be streaked with blood
Abdominal distension
Dryness of the throat
Nervous tension
Hiccups
Nausea
Burning sensation in the stomach

Sweet foods, over-consumption of.

Thin eyebrows or no eyebrows at all
Palm of the hand blue or purple
White spots on the nails
White nails

Tetanus.

Rigid contractions in neck and jaw
Chills
Headaches
Swallowing becomes difficult

Teeth grit together
Becomes physically weaker

Thyroid trouble.
Bulging eyes
Swollen eyelids
Swollen face
Loss of hair
Feeling the cold all the time
No energy and constant fatigue
Lack of appetite

Tonsilitis.
Sore and painful throat
Tonsils swollen
Ulcers may develop on the tonsils
Yellow patches appear on the tonsils
Sometimes the throat swells
Occasional chills or fever
Convulsions are possible
Throat is red

Trachoma.
Spots inside the eyelid
Upper eyelid swollen and hard
Blurred vision
Increased eye secretion
Itching eye

Tuberculosis.
Cheeks turn pink in the afternoon
Thick yellow sputum
Frequent urination; and urine dark yellow
Abdomen soft and painful to the touch
Sometimes bright red blood is vomited
Reddish tongue
White fur on the tongue
Feverish hands and feet
Night sweats
Tiredness

Dry mouth and throat, and constantly thirsty
Dry stools
Mentally depressed

Tumours.
Dark gums and lips
Cysts on the lips
Tarry stolls
Swollen abdomen
Poor appetite
Belching
Pains in chest, abdomen or back
Acid taste to the sputum
Nausea
Dramatic weight loss
Frequent headaches
Anaemia
Women may show blood in the discharge
Skin adopts an orange-green hue
Jaundice
Blood streaks the motions
Very fatigued

Urine infection.
Frequent urination, which may be painful
Urine may sometimes contain gravel
Variations in quantity of urine
Face may turn yellow
Fatigue
Loss of weight
Thirstiness
Bladder tender to touch
Enlarged prostate
Headaches
Dark-coloured urine

Urine retention.
Severe swelling of the abdomen
Cannot pass any urine, or only a few drops at a time
Navel and feet are cold to the touch

Feverish
Delirious
Fur on tongue either thin and white or thick and yellow
Nervousness

Jrticaria.
White or pink weals appear on the skin
Severe itching at spasmodic times, especially at night
After scratching the weals swell up into bumps
Nausea
Abdominal pains
Dry, itchy throat
Diarrhoea
Constipation
Tense and apprehensive
White or yellow fur on the tongue
Pink tongue
Parasites in the motion

Jterus trouble.
Heel of the palm dark red
Weakness
Yellow urine
Backache
Yellow fur on tongue
Pale tongue
Frequent urination
Thin and loose stools

Vaste matter, an excess in the system.
White or yellow moles on the tongue
Red pimples on the body
Red rashes on the body
Red palms and fingers

Vhooping Cough.
Smooth white sputum
Runny nose
Sneezing
Hard hacking cough

Minute ulcers at the base of the tongue
Fever
Vomiting, which may contain blood
Blue complexion
Bloodshot eyes
Very pale fingertips
Pale lips
White or yellow fur on the tongue
Pink tongue
Dry mouth

Worms and parasites.
Concave nails
Hard and cracked nails
Frequent nail-biting
Rectal irritation
Abdominal pain
Swollen abdomen
White blotches on the face
Blue or purple specks on eyeballs
Nausea
Dizziness
Fever
Skin rash
Small red spots on the tongue and behind the lower lip
Putrid smell to the motion
Pale complexion
Weariness
Itching round the anus and sometimes the vagina

Yin foods, over-consumption of.
Dark lips
Dark blue or purple palms
White nails
Pale, white, glossy and transparent complexion
Red blotches on the skin
Skin cold and damp, especially hands and feet

Chapter 8

Study your own Pulse

As we have seen all illnesses are made by man himself, and are caused through the disturbance of the body energies, which in turn disturbs the balance between the Yin and Yang within the human anatomy. Whilst this tipping of the scales, either too much one way or the other, is largely due to the bad eating and drinking habits, or to numerous drugs and medicaments, or the quantities of chemicals in packaged and tin foods, it can also be influenced through excessive cold or heat and strong emotional upsets like anger, hate or fear.

Generally however, if the body is truly healthy, and constantly retains the proper balance within itself, so that the natural phenomenal changes can take effect at the proper times of the day or night, and the energy levels of the various organs can be correctly maintained during the course of each day, then even excess emotions will have little or no effect, for the body and the mind will be strong enough to cope with it at any time.

Let us take the situation of Cathy who had suffered terrible family upsets, lasting over many months, and her health had deteriorated so far that she had twice tried to commit suicide. A close friend was so worried that she might try again that she sought help from her nearest Ch'ang Ming adviser. Cathy was willing to try altering her complete way of life, and, by strictly adhering to the diet prescribed for her, her health improved so much that it was better than it had ever been before, and she was able to face her family problems with resolution and courage. The same problems still exist, but she handles them with fortitude and confidence. She has become one with herself, and also has become an integral part of nature, a true child of the universe.

For thousands of years the Chinese have known that there was a very close relationship between the heartbeat (Yang), rate of breathing (Yin), energy flow (Yang) and blood flow (Yin), and all these gave the state of a person's overall health, and the efficiency of his organs. All these are still used in Chinese diagnosis, and the pulse is an extremely important indicator of the health.

To the average Westerner, "feeling the pulse" means no more than placing one finger on an artery, generally at the wrist, to feel it pulsating. This is caused by the rhythmic pulsation of the heart as the blood is pumped out of the left ventricle and, owing to the force of the flow, distends the walls of the aorta, so creating the vibrations that in turn produce the pulsating of the arteries. By counting the number of pulsations, one can tell whether the heart is beating at the right rate, too slow or too fast. Generally speaking, a man's heart should beat between sixty-four and seventy-two times a minute, while a woman's should beat between seventy-two and eighty times a minute.

Chinese medical practitioners take the pulse not only at the wrist, but also, if necessary, at the arteries of the neck and legs, and several other places where an artery is close to a bone and near to the surface of the skin. This is because the pulse can provide a wealth of information about the condition of the organs of the human body, and not just an indication of the body's general health. Through the pulse the energy level of each organ can be judged, and thus whether the organ is working properly, erratically, congested, too full, deficient, slippery, rapid, solid or empty. The experienced Chinese physician can tell from the pulse the patient's health history and what his future health is likely to be if he does not change his way of life.

You too can learn how to obtain such information by "feeling" and "reading" your own pulse. There is nothing difficult about it; all you have to do is concentrate on the "feel" of the pulse, so as to be able to understand what it can convey. In China we have to learn to read our own pulse before we can practise the art on others, and if we are going to be a healer of any kind, then we must set an example, by being healthy and fit ourselves.

In any case, wouldn't it be a wonderful thing to understand and appreciate the standard of your own internal health and the fluctuations of energy that take place within each organ at various times of the day. You will also have the pleasure of being able to help your relations and friends, when called upon to do so, and be in a position to give them a deeper insight to their problems.

In ancient China you never had to pay the doctor when you were ill, because you were unable to perform your daily work, so naturally you were in no position to earn any money, and there were no state benefits in those days. So you paid your doctor to keep you well and fit whilst you were well enough to earn a living, so it was his responsibility to ensure that you were healthy all the time. If this standard was adopted in the Western world what an enormous saving there would be in National Health Services.

The Nei Ching, the Yellow Emperor's Classic of Internal Medicine, specifies that the best time of the day to take the pulse is early in the morning, before the Yang part of the day has begun and the Yin section has started to fail, and before any food or drink had been consumed, before the twelve organs have become invigorated, and while the energy levels have not yet reached their peak or had been extended. The seasons too were said to influence the pulse to a considerable degree, and it was even recommended that the physician calculate the astrologically most favourable moment to take his patient's pulse. All this may seem to you very complicated, but it will convey the meticulousness of the ancient Chinese doctor in caring for his patients, and in seeking an absolute correct diagnosis.

The pulse can, however, be read at any time, and this is how you should do it. First of all, sit down and relax completely. Next place your left forearm across your chest and rest your right palm against the back of your left wrist; then curl the fingers of your right hand round your left wrist, and you will find that your index finger is at the base of your left palm, below the thumb. You will feel a pulsation with your right index finger, and this will tell you that you are in contact with the radial artery of your left wrist. Place the middle finger of your right hand alongside your index finger, and allow your third or "ring" finger to rest close to your middle finger, so that the three fingers are close together. Next press one finger at a time gently down on to the radial artery, and in each case you will feel a pulsation with the tip of the finger.

Practise this as many times a day as you can, and whenever you can find the time, and you will begin to notice that there are slight variations in what you can feel at each finger tip. If you practise at the same times each day, then you will get a clearer understanding of the differences, until eventually you are able to read your pulse as easily as reading a book.

Don't become anxious if the pulse feels stronger at one point

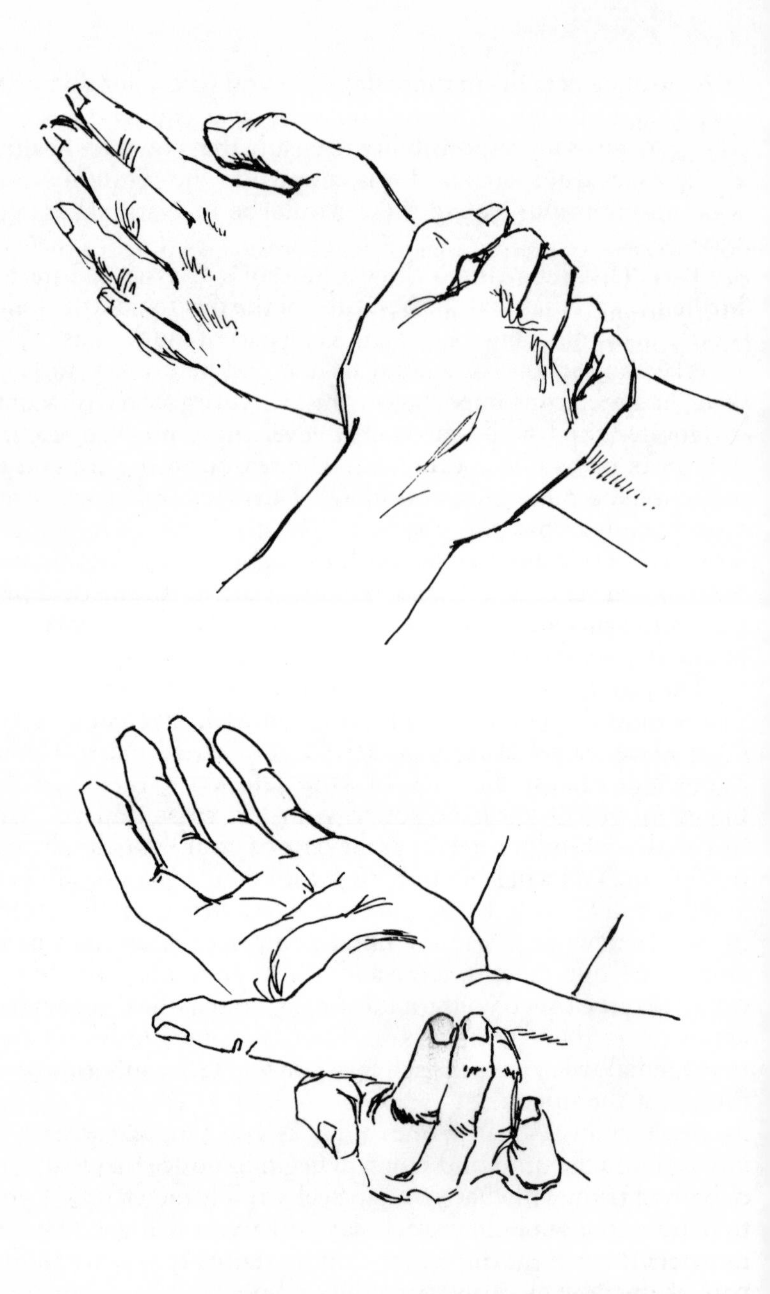

than another, for remember that all organs have their peak periods and low phases, and this will effect a difference in what you can feel, through the pulsations underneath your finger tips.

Give yourself time, and practise continuously, and interpretation will slowly come to you. Remember, that the pulse of both wrists can be felt, but to begin with only practise on one side first. The organs about which your left radial artery conveys information to you are different from those you can learn about from your right radial artery.

What does this mean? Simply this, that there are two levels of pressure with each of the finger tips, a light or superficial touch or a strong or deep pressure, which gives six different pulses on each wrist, making a total of twelve pulses in all, each separate pulse giving the condition of a different organ within the body.

	Yang organs *Slight pressure*	*Yin organs* *Strong pressure*
Left radial artery (left wrist)		
Tip of index finger	Small intestine	Heart
Tip of middle finger	Gall bladder	Liver
Tip of third finger	Urinary bladder	Kidneys
Right radial artery (right wrist)		
Tip of index finger	Large intestine	Lungs
Tip of middle finger	Stomach	Spleen
Tip of third Finger	"Triple warmer"	"Heart controller"

You will recognise all these organs with the possible exception of the last two, the Triple warmer and the Heart controller, which we will explain to you so that you will have a better understanding of their sphere of influence.

The "triple warmer" known also as the "triple heater", "three burning spheres", and "heat regulator", is not connected to any specific organ of the body. It regulates the changes, indicates variations of temperature, and the operational effects of both of them within the human body. It is extremely sensitive to minute changes in the body's internal temperature relative to its external temperature, and to the transfer of energy from one part of the body to another. It also controls the quantity and quality of waste products in the system; and indirectly it is the functional overlord of the digestion and ingestion, and of the dissipation and utilization of heat within the body; which taking drugs of any kind can radically upset. It thus has a very big job to do; and you can gauge how well it is performing by exerting a slight pressure on the right wrist with tip of the third finger of the left hand. (Triple warmer trouble is also indicated by a moon at the top of the iris.)

If you press strongly with the same finger on the same artery, you will then be feeling the variations in the "heart controller", also known as the "controller of the heart", "heart governor" or "circulation path", which relates to the circulation of the body. Like the "triple warmer" it is not connected or linked to any specific organ of the body, but it represents the functional system of the arteries, veins and the circulation of the blood throughout the entire human body. It controls the distribution of the blood and other fluids in the blood-stream, whether it is oxygenated or not. It also arranges the nourishment of all the Yin organs of the body.

What of the other organs, such as the heart, liver, kidneys, intestines, etc., and what do we expect to extract from the delicate touch, and the sense or feel of the vibrations of each separate pulse. Every organ has an energy level, activated and constantly maintains through your food intake and your breathing, and this nutrition and respiration converts eventually into physical energy and internal energy. These energies are distributed throughout the whole body and inhabit every tissue and cell, and through the pulse you will be able to judge the strength or weakness of them in the various organs, and, thus, how healthy those organs are.

The pulse of a normal healthy person is firm and regular, and it should beat at the rate of four times to each intake of breath. But how do we categorise the various differences that are felt so that an accurate diagnosis can be made. Simply, all the classifications fall into Yin and Yang sections.

Yang pulses.

1 Floating—a very light sensation, almost as if the pulse was floating under the skin and it indicates an external deficiency.

2 Rapid—a very rapid pulsation denoting a hot disease.
3 Solid—a forceful beat showing a solid type of illness such as abdominal upsets, constipation and urinary troubles.
4 Full—long and hard with a feeling of tightness generally felt in people who are suffering from internal pain or liver disease.

Yin pulses.

5 Sunken—felt as a forceful pulse but only under heavy pressure and shows that there is an internal deficiency.
6 Slow—less than four beats to one breath and indicates an aversion to cold temperature, as well as suffering from cold hands, feet and complexion.
7 Deficient—weak pulsation under light or heavy pressure and denotes a general weakness caused by the lack of blood and energy.
8 Slippery—the pulse feels very smooth and is generally seen in people who tend to emit a lot of mucus, and who may suffer from palpitations. It may also be felt in women who are pregnant.

So through feeling the pulse you acquire the experience of being able to define the various differences in the rhythm, slow or fast, whether it is weak or strong, normal or abnormal, smooth as silk or irregular and bumpy. Admittedly, it will take time to acquire the "feel" of the touch and to interpret the differences skilfully.

Persevere, and you will be amazed at the sensitivity you acquire to the changes that take place within the body. This is one sure way of identifying any weaknesses that may occur, even before there is any outward symptom of their existence, so that you may, in accordance with the supreme laws of the universe, correct them before it is too late. By this means constant good health and adequate vitality may be assured.

Chapter 9

Nutrition

Food is the life-line of the body. Eat the right foods and you guarantee yourself constant good health for the rest of your life; eat the wrong foods and you deplete your reserves of energy, over-work the organs of the body, and so commit yourself to illness. The choice is between the Yin, and decline, and the Yang, and good health.

If you are not eating the right things at the moment, then, regardless of whether or not you are now ill, you would be wise to change your habits and try to live according to the laws of nature. Good health can be obtained only through a proper diet and not through drugs and medicines, which can eradicate the symptoms but not the cause, and may have undesirable side-effects. Again, the choice is between the Yin and the Yang.

A great many people are already fully aware of the benefits of Ch'ang Ming and have discovered the benefit of correct eating and drinking habits to the physical side of their lives, and, through that, to their spiritual growth. So that others, too, may appreciate the importance of a correct diet, this chapter examines the nutritional needs of the body and how they can be satisfied.

Proteins

Proteins must be an integral part of the daily diet, for they provide the basis for the growth of all living tissue and for its repair. All proteins are broken down into amino-acids through digestion; these contain carbon, hydrogen, oxygen, nitrogen, sulphur and sometimes phosphorus, and can assume an infinite variety of combinations.

Many vegetable foods, including grains, peas, beans, nuts, seeds, soya beans, root vegetables, and many leafy greens, contain amino-acids, but a mixed diet of grains and good vegetables (preferably organically grown) is particularly beneficial. It is well known that in some vegetables there is a greater amount of amino-acids than in meat, and, as a result, vegetarians will tend to gain more essential goodness from their food, and to heal more quickly of an injury, than do non-vegetarians. Added to this, by not eating meat the risk of side effects is considerably reduced.

Animal protein is obtained from lean meat, fish, liver, milk, cheese and eggs, but, because the stomach takes so long to digest them, bacteria develop and poisons are produced and this places a strain on the organs of the body. So, while animal protein has a biological value, its goodness is counter-balanced by the harmful waste that ensues from its consumption, and it is best to exclude it from the diet.

Unfortunately, animo-acids surplus to needs cannot be stored in the human body, so sensible eating habits are essential if the body is to have the correct intake of protein at all times.

Vitamins

Vitamins are highly complex organic substances that occur in very small quantities in the food, and each has a special job of work to do in ensuring that a particular organ or a group of organs functions properly and that good health is secured. Unfortunately, the human body cannot make vitamins, and the only way in which these necessities can be obtained is through the diet.

However, it has been proved that excessive use of vitamin tablets has very little effect, as most of the intake disappears into the urine. What is essential is that there should be a proper balance of vitamins and minerals within the body. Deficiencies in this respect can cause ill health and restrict growth, especially in children.

Vitamins fall into two main groups: those that are easily dissolved in water but are not affected by fat or oil (water-soluble) and those that dissolve in fat and oils but are unaffected in water (fat-soluble). Thus, proper cooking is essential if the vitamins in food are not to be destroyed.

Vitamin A is essential for the vision and for the constant growth of healthy skin tissue; it assists in the protection of the body against infection; it repairs internal or external weaknesses; and it is stored in the liver. Excess heat will not normally affect it, but air has a tendency to make it unstable.

A healthy skin is always moist to the touch; and, because Vitamin A is fat-soluble, normal washing will not remove it. If, however, the skin becomes dry and scaly, there is a deficiency of the vitamin.

Lack of Vitamin A can cause night blindness, which is the condition where a person has extreme difficulty in seeing properly in dim light or at night time, although during the day the vision appears to be normal. The purple (rhodopsin) which should be present in the rods of the retina, and allows us to see in darkness, is directly derived from this vitamin. Every year, thousands of children in the poor countries of the world go blind owing to an infection (keratomalacia) caused by a deficiency of Vitamin A.

Vitamin A will combat infection in the urinary and respiratory tracts, but lack of it can cause the formation of gallbladder and kidney stones, and weaknesses in respiration (which will show up in constant coughs and colds, sinus troubles and catarrh). Important sources of Vitamin A are:

vegetables — broccoli, cabbage, peas, watercress, carrots, spinach, kale, asparagus, alfalfa, turnip greens, beet greens, mustard greens, pumpkins, dandelion greens and tomatoes;
fruits — apricots, yellow peaches;
animal sources — liver, halibut-liver oil, cod-liver oil, margarine, butter, egg yolks, Cheddar cheese.

Potatoes do not contain any Vitamin A.

Vitamin B. The B group of vitamins is very large and includes thiamine (Vitamin B_1); riboflavin, nictonic acid, pyridoxine, pantothenic acid, biotin, inositol and folic acid (all vitamins of the B_2 complex) and cyanocobalamin (Vitamin B_{12}). Although these vitamins differ from each other in their chemical structure, they have many features in common. For instance, they are all water-soluble, they come from the same type of foods, and none of them can be stored for very long in the body, which means that there needs to be a regular daily intake of them.

Overcooking or boiling in too much water can entirely destroy these vital vitamins, so one way of obtaining them is to eat the foods uncooked. If cooking is necessary or preferred, sautéing is the best method. Pasteurisation partially destroys the B vitamins, and ultra-violet light and water that is too acid or too alkaline may have the same effects.

The B vitamins are stored in the liver. They help to stimulate the appetite, aid digestion, promote growth through the goodness in the bloodstream and in turn through the bone marrow, aid the functioning of the nervous system, and increase energy and resistance against infection.

Lack of these vitamins can result in beri-beri, which is generally caused by eating only polished rice (in the Second World War it was very common among prisoners of the Japanese) but may also be caused by an excessive intake of alcohol. Deficiency of B vitamins can also cause digestive, intestinal and gastric malfunctions, brain troubles (such as delirium), fevers, poor memory, nervousness, schizophrenia, and lack of awareness and concentration. It can also show up in the form of skin complaints, such as dermatitis and eczema, and in the fact that the slightest scratch or graze on the skin may become inflamed or infected.

The B vitamins can be found in:

grains, vegetables, etc. — wheat, millet, rye, brown rice, oatmeal, cornflakes, soya beans, kelp, sunflower seeds, sesame seeds, green leafy vegetables, peas, beans, almonds, roasted peanuts, lentils and yeast extracts;
animal sources — fish, chicken, eggs, Cheddar cheese, liver, beef, lamb, pork and milk.

Potatoes and beer contain minute amounts of these vitamins.

Thiamine (Vitamin B_1). Thiamine is absolutely necessary for the release of energy from carbohydrates in the diet, and lack of it will result in beri-beri. Fats, sugar and beer contain no thiamine whatsoever.

Wheat is a major source of it, but in the preparation of white flour most of it is removed with the bran in the milling process. It is best, then, to eat wholemeal bread, in which the thiamine is retained in its natural state.

In addition to wheat, other grains contain thiamine, and so do vegetables, kelp, almonds, roasted peanuts, soya beans, lentils, brown rice, beans and peas.

Riboflavin is water-soluble and very stable in heat; but alkaline substances and ultra-violet light are highly detrimental to it. It is bright yellow and is easily stored in the body.

Riboflavin is essential for the utilisation of energy from the food we eat, for it converts foods into protein and derives iron from other minerals; and it is necessary for healthy skin tissue and good vision. Lack of it restricts growth, reduces the health of skin tissue and causes loss of hair, eye troubles (sometimes cataracts), a general lack of energy, ulcers on the tongue, and sores in the corners of the mouth. Good sources of this vitamin are:

vegetables, etc. — cabbage, carrots, watercress, spinach, turnip greens, dandelion greens, grains, prunes, apples, apricots, coconuts and yeast extract;
animal sources — liver, kidneys, eggs, Cheddar cheese, chicken, beef and milk.

Potatoes contain a negligible amount.

Nicotinic acid (niacin) and nicotinamide are involved in utilising energy from food, and lack of them results in a disease known as pellagra, which was once found in places where maize was the main diet, but is now also found in people who suffer from chronic digestive disorders and whose diet is extremely poor, so preventing them from absorbing the vitamins (chronic alcoholics can suffer this disease.). The symptoms are diarrhoea, mental illness and dermatitis.

The curious fact about nicotinic acid is that in some foods it occurs in a bound form and therefore is unavailable to the digestive system of man, while in some foods (for instance, eggs and milk) that do not contain it an amino-acid called tryptophan is present, and this the body can convert into nicotinic acid. It is present in, or may be derived from, the following foods:

vegetables, etc. — grains, peas and beans;

animal sources — white fish, chicken, eggs, Cheddar cheese, pork, beef, milk.

Pyridoxine is necessary in the production of haemoglobin (the oxygen-carrying pigment in the red blood cells), in the conversion of tryptophan into nicotinic acid, and so on. Women who are pregnant and who are not eating sensibly could suffer a deficiency which could affect the child they are carrying: and women who are taking birth-control pills will generally be deficient in this very important vitamin.

Pyridoxine is found in many foods, especially in grains, most vegetables, fish, eggs and meat.

Pantothenic acid. This one vitamin that man does not have to worry about too much for it is so prevalent in his diet that he can hardly fail to get adequate supplies. Its main task is to release energy from fats and carbohydrates. Grains, peas, beans and seeds are particularly rich sources of this vitamin.

Biotin is essential for the metamorphosis of fat, but such small amounts of it are needed by the body as generally to cause no worries. However, if a large number of raw eggs are swallowed, the biotin in the body may be eliminated. Sources of biotin are grains, vegetables, fruit, egg yolks, milk and offal.

Folic acid has many functions, and one of the main ones is its interaction with cyanocobalamin (vitamin B_{12}). Deficiency can be caused through alcoholism, pregnancy, giving birth prematurely, drugs, and, in elderly people, especially by poor diets.

Cyanocobalamin (Vitamin B_{12}) is a composition of several compounds, which contain particles of cobalt. With folic acid, it helps many cells in the body, particularly in the bone marrow. Deficiency of it can lead to deterioration of the nerve cells and to pernicious anaemia. Sources of this vitamin are white fish, eggs, Cheddar cheese, yeast extract, beef, lamb and pork, but the richest source of it is liver.

Vitamin C (ascorbic acid). Man is one of the few creatures that cannot make its own Vitamic C, and so he must obtain it through his diet. He obtains it mostly from fruit and vegetables. The richest sources of it are rose hips, blackcurrants, soya beans and sprouts, and it is an interesting fact that soya beans and sprouts, when put into a refrigerator, increase their Vitamin C content. Unfortunately, the body stores very little of it and so it is essential that it is consumed daily. It needs to be remembered, however, that it is water-soluble and that ordinary cooking methods largely destroy it. For this reason, the best cooking methods to use are sautéing and steam cooking.

Vitamic C helps to fight infection, keeps the veins and capillaries in a good condition, and also maintains the health of the skin tissues. One of the first signs of a deficiency of it is bleeding gums, but it can also show up through a shortage of breath, scurvy, teeth trouble, increased heart action, tender joints and ulcers.

Most people are under the impression that to gain plenty of Vitamin C they should eat more oranges and lemons, but you get at least a third more of this vital vitamin by eating Brussels sprouts, cauliflower and cabbage.

Vitamin D. The greatest source of this is sunlight on the skin, which is more than adequate for the average person, but other rich sources are herrings, kippers, sardines, margarine and cod-liver oil.

Vitamin D is soluble in fats and oils, but insoluble in water, it regulates the utilisation of calcium and phosphorus to make strong bones and teeth, and a lack of it can cause rickets in children and deformation in adults (in particular, bowlegs, triangular pelvis, bent spine, and swollen elbows and wrists).

Vitamin E (tocopherol) is derived mainly from wheatgerm oil, but is also found in parsley, spinach, lettuce, celery and watercress and to a lesser degree in cereals and egg yolk. It is fat-soluble and ordinary light has no effect upon it, though ultraviolet light can gradually diminish its effectiveness.

Lack of this vitamin has been proved to cause infertility in rats, and it is suspected that it also causes sterility in humans. The vitamin is of benefit to the blood vessels and the heart, and, because it is stored mainly in the muscle fibres, is generally used very quickly, and so needs continual replacement.

Vitamin K is necessary for the normal clotting of the blood and is synthesised by bacteria in the bowels. Unless there is a disease of the intestines or the liver, a deficiency of the vitamin is most unlikely, as it can be found in all vegetables (especially spinach, cabbage, cauliflower and peas) and in grains, and egg yolk.

Minerals

There are at least twenty minerals or elements within the human body, and it is generally recognised that fifteen of them are absolutely essential. The main functions of minerals are threefold:

1 to form bones and teeth;
2 to assist in controlling the composition of fluids and cells within the body;
3 to act with enzymes and proteins in the release and utilisation of energy.

Of the fifteen minerals that are considered really essential to the health of the body, those that are needed in the largest amounts are calcium, phosphorus, sulphur, potassium, sodium, chlorine, magnesium, and iron, and the other seven are required in such minute quantities that they are generally referred to as trace elements.

Calcium is absorbed from the intestines and aids in the utilisation of Vitamin D to make strong bones and teeth. It is also required for the proper clotting of the blood; for the benefit of the heart, the muscles and the nerves; and to reduce fatigue and increase stamina and mental alertness. Lack of it is a cause of rickets, osteomalacia, contraction of the muscles, brittle nails, fits and other mental disorders, skin complaints and dry hair. Women have a tendency to lose large quantities of calcium when they bear children in fairly quick succession and they also lose quite a lot when they breast-feed their babies. For the benefit not only of themselves but also of their babies, it is essential that this loss is made good. Growing children too need extra quantities of calcium, as their bones grow and they develop new teeth.

In a normal diet, only about 25 per cent of the calcium is utilised by the body, and even this percentage is dependent on the amount of Vitamin D that has been absorbed. The remainder is lost in the motions of the bowels. To obtain as much calcium as possible, the following foods (listed in descending order of the amount of calcium they contain) should be included in the diet: powdered dried skimmed milk, Cheddar cheese, tinned sardines, watercress, cabbage, grains, eggs and white fish.

Iron is present in the haemoglobin in the red blood corpuscles, which have a life-span of about three to four months. Their iron content is not wasted, for the body efficiently reutilises it, but if there is not sufficient iron in the diet the body's reserves of it become depleted, the body draws on the iron in the haemoglobin, and anemia results. Sources of iron include:

vegetables, etc. — grains, watercress, peas, beans, turnips, carrots, dates, prunes, raisins, figs and bananas;
animal sources — liver, kidney, beef, chicken and white fish.

Phosphorus, next to calcium, is the most prominent mineral in the human body. It is a major constituent of every living cell and it helps in obtaining energy from the food consumed. In harmony with calcium it ensures that bones and teeth gain strength. It is an important part of many acids and fats, carbohydrates and proteins, and combines with Vitamins A, C, D and some B to activate them. Sometimes the urine takes on a cloudy appearance, which indicates that excess phosphates are being discharged; this is no cause for alarm, for a deficiency is almost unknown (it can occur if rat poison is swallowed; this causes liver damage and acts as an irritant). Phosphorus is present in all grain foods, seeds, most vegetables and many fruits.

Potassium is largely found within the fluids of the body cells, and excess quantities are excreted through the kidneys. Diuretics and purgatives, if taken too frequently, can cause potassium deficiencies, and even vomiting and diarrhoea can result in a loss.

A severe lack of potassium can cause thirstiness and giddiness and can also affect the muscles, including those of the heart. Heart failure may result.

Nearly all grains, seeds, vegetables and fruits supply enough of this mineral for the requirements of the human body.

Sodium is essential to the muscles and nervous system and to the fluids outside the body cells, such as saliva, the digestive juices and bile. It helps to maintain the fluid balance. Lack of it can lead to muscular cramps, fainting and dizziness, and an excess to kidney upsets and high blood pressure.

Some of the best sources of supply of sodium are:

vegetables, grains, etc. — whole wheat, cornflakes, rye, watercress, spinach, peas, beans, dandelion greens and prunes;
animal sources — haddock, herrings (including kippers), chicken, bacon, kidney and margarine.

Magnesium strengthens the bones and teeth, the tissues and the nervous system, and assists in obtaining energy from food. Deficiency of it is very rare, because it is present in most foods; but chronic diarrhoea can eliminate the body supply and thereby create depressions, fatigue and convulsions. The best sources of magnesium are yeast extract, roasted peanuts, grains, chicken and Cheddar cheese, and it is present in most vegetables.

Sulphur. Most foods contain sulphur, and the best from a nutritional point of view are grains, vegetables, fruit, eggs and nuts. Sulphur is found within the cells of the tissues and therefore acts within the skin and the bones; it helps to cleanse the blood and reduce toxin accumulation. A deficiency can lead to the diseases normally associated with uric acid and the side effects it has on the system.

Chlorine is an essential constituent of the body fluid and works in close harmony with sodium as a cleanser of the blood, for it helps to eradicate harmful bacteria. It also reduces unnecessary fat in the tissues. Whilst the chlorine content of most foods is comparatively low, most grains, fruits and vegetables contain small quantities, and the use of sea salt will help, especially in cases where there is excessive perspiration.

Trace elements. These include iodine, cobalt, copper,

chromium, fluorine, manganese and zinc. Most of them play only a small role, and so it is very difficult to tell exactly what effect they have on each other, how the body utilises them, and what their role is. Iodine, however, is an exception, for it is essential to the hormones, which are produced by the thyroid gland (in the neck), and a deficiency of it causes goitre. Whilst grains and vegetables contain minute amounts, depending on the type of soil in which they grow, the greatest source of iodine is seafood, especially seaweed. In China, unless you are a very long way from the coast, goitre is almost unknown, because seaweed is regularly eaten as a vegetable. If you find it hard to obtain, then the next best thing is kelp, obtainable from most health shops.

Chapter 10

Ch'ang Ming is long life

It is an old saying in China that "Old age is inevitable, but there is no excuse for senility". As we have already seen, illness is absolutely unnecessary, and is caused by bad eating and drinking habits. In China, where the normal diet is much healthier than in the West, many of the illnesses most prevalent in the West are scarcely known.

Ch'ang Ming, the Taoist Long Life therapy has played an important part in Chinese eating and drinking habits for thousands of years. Derived from the basic principles laid down by the "Sons of Reflected Light", which are incorporated in the foundations of the "Five Elements" in reference to the Yin and Yang aspects affecting the human body, it has been handed down from family to family throughout the vast expanse of China, and has become a natural part of the average family way of living, so that it is now second nature to them.

Most people never think of their health while it remains reasonably sound, but they may be so abusing it in so many different ways that sooner or later the system is bound to break down and succumb to illness. The vitality of youth may conceal physical weaknesses, and if a child does complain continuously about various aches and pains and other upsets it is usually put down to "growing pains". As age takes its normal course through life, then degeneration and the natural deterioration that goes with it starts to take place, and it is then that the real weaknesses within the framework of their physical structure starts to become more and more noticeable. The body, not having the necessary strength to fight back, will slowly wilt under the strain and become racked with illnesses. If you allow the foundations, the walls, and the roof of your house to deteriorate, then eventually it will collapse and you will have nothing left but a pile of useless rubble.

That is exactly what many people in the West do to their own bodies, and then they wonder what has gone wrong, and put the blame everywhere but on themselves, which is where it belongs. We will give you a good guideline to good health—if you catch one cold or lose your temper once in your lifetime, then you are sick, and you must do something about it AT ONCE.

There is no excuse for undermining the health of the human body, the most wondrous creation of the Supreme Spirit. Perfect in every detail, with working parts that replace themselves constantly, built-in thermostats to guard against the cold and changes in the atmosphere, an automatic cooling system that refreshes you in the extreme heat, and essential organs that work for twenty-four hours every day and never go on strike, unless you overload them, and they all do their own particular jobs to the very best of their ability without thanks or recompense.

No engineer could ever design a machine that could do the same job over and over again throughout such a long period of time, no heating expert has ever devised such a marvellous automatic system, and look at the wonderful way everything within this physical structure, called the human body, can not only look after itself, arrange its own maintenance, but also renew its own parts.

It has within itself a huge work-force, which it feeds, houses, and, if they die, replaces them at very short notice. It has the most efficient power and sewerage systems ever designed. This wonder of wonders, this miracle of miracles, this treasure beyond all treasures, and yet, many constantly abuse it every day. Sending the workers on strike, killing off the army of protectors, severely overloading the power and sewerage systems, and packing out the warehouses with useless rubbish, so that there is no space left for the essentials.

If you owned the greatest treasure in the world, what would you do? You would make sure that it was fully protected in every possible way, you would see that it was kept at the right temperature, regularly cleaned every day so that its beauty could be admired by everyone, and you would be proud to put it on show for the whole world to see.

Well, you do own the greatest treasure in the world; it was given to you by the will of the Tao, and you gained possession of it in your mother's uterus, so why not be sensible and learn to guard and protect it properly every day of your life, wrap it up well in the cold and help to keep the warmth in, just as you lag your water tanks, and give it air when it's hot, just as you open the windows of your home to let the air circulate. Then you will be able to tell the world what a wonderful treasure you own, and show it off with pride.

Ch'ang Ming is based on very sound biological principles, proved and tested over 10,000 years of history. The early Taoists, recognising that "the proof of the pudding is in the eating", used their own bodies to test it over many centuries, sometimes eating only brown rice, sometimes only meat, at other times only fruit, during other periods only seafood, and so on. No other art has been so thoroughly proved, and no medical organisation has practised their knowledge and skill over such a long period. So that today millions enjoy the benefits of Ch'ang Ming, which is based on just a few simple rules:

1 Eat only when hungry, and not just out of habit.
2 Eat only natural foods.
3 Eat more grains and vegetables.
4 Chew all your food really well.
5 Don't over-eat at any time.
6 Keep your liquid intake down to the barest minimum.
7 Take deep breaths whenever you get the opportunity.

Because Ch'ang Ming was based on such simple rules it became necessary to know the fundamental biological foundations of all food that was grown, plant, flower, fruit, root, and all other living matter, and to understand what long term effect each one had upon the human body. So it came to be that after 10,000 years of study and practice, practitioners of this art in China had a very deep insight and understanding of the laws and principles of the universe, and they were all very competent dieticians and herbalists, based on the Taoist experimentations on themselves in their search for physical and spiritual alchemy.

Naturally, Chinese herbal therapy (Ts'ao Yao) is an intimate companion of Ch'ang Ming, and together they have led to some wonderful discoveries, not only in the field of plant life, but also in the area of minerals, ores and liquids. Did you know that the shell of the tortoise can be used to cure malaria and infantile convulsions, that your own hair, when carbonised, can stop a nosebleed, that the centipede is good against lockjaw and snake-bites, that the poison in potatoes can help cure arthritis, and that pepper, when used as a medicine, can cure dysentry and food-poisoning? Chinese herbal therapy details thousands of recipes for health, but they would not be needed if everyone learnt to eat and drink sensibly, and in accordance with the laws of nature.

Nearly sixty years ago, Chan Kam Lee, in all his illustrious wisdom, allied the Taoist rules and recommendations to foods and drinks normally consumed in the West, and, by balancing the Yin and Yang intake, came up with the following suggestions:

Ch'ang Ming health diet

Foods that are NOT to be eaten

1 Refined and processed foods. If any colourings, preservatives, flavourings, or other chemicals are included, don't touch it.
2 Any grain foods that has been processed, especially white bread and anything made from white flour.
3 All deep fried foods.
4 Coffee, alcohol, tobacco, chocolate and other sweets.
5 Spices, rock salt, mustard, pepper, vinegar, pickles, curry.
6 Meat such as pork, beef, mutton and lamb.
7 Salmon, mackerel, shark, swordfish, tuna and whale.
8 Sugar.
9 Ice cream, artificial jellies, synthetic fruit juices.
10 Potatoes, tomatoes, aubergines, rhubarb, spinach.
11 Concentrated meat extracts, soups and gravies.
12 Milk, cheese, butter, dairy yoghurt, boiled or fried eggs.
13 Lard or dripping that comes from animal fats.
14 Any bird or fish that has a lot of fat tissue.

Foods that may be eaten.

1 Anything made from natural whole grain, that has not been refined, e.g. brown rice, buckwheat, wheat, barley, millet, rye, maize and includes bread, cakes, puddings, biscuits, breakfast foods etc.
2 All locally grown vegetables that are in season, especially root vegetables, excluding those items in previous list, No. 10.

3 Soya-bean and mung-bean shoots.
4 Seaweed.
5 Locally grown fruit and berries (moderately).
6 Nuts, preferably roasted—but not salted.
7 Low fat natural yoghurt.
8 Honey (sparingly).
9 Cottage cheese or vegetarian cheese.
10 Herb teas and China teas.
11 Vegetable margarine and oils (e.g. sesame, sunflower, safflower).
12 Eggs, but only scrambled or in omelettes—better still eat the yolks only.
13 Natural sea salt, sesame seed salt, soya sauce.
14 All dried fruits—cherries, raisins, currants etc.
15 All grain milks, rice milk and coconut milk.
16 Wild vegetables and herbs.
17 Fruit drinks made from locally grown fresh fruit—ideally, make your own.

Utilise the following, if necessary.
18 Non-fat fish excluding those in previous list, No. 7.
19 Sea-food—shrimps, prawns etc. But be wary of crab.
20 Wild birds—pheasant, pigeon etc.
21 Wild or free range chicken, turkey etc.
22 Skimmed milk or powdered skimmed milk.

The average Chinese has only two meals a day, and over the entire history of China this has been found perfectly adequate. This enables the body to digest the food intake from one meal, to distribute it properly about the system, and then have sufficient time to rest until the next intake of food.

Now what are natural foods? Mention natural foods to the average person and they will immediately think that you are a quack or a faddist, but in so doing, they have over-looked the fact that natural food has been the life line of humanity for thousands of years, and it is only in the last few decades that chemicals have become more widely used in pesticides, fertilisers, bleaches, additives, colourings, preservatives, flavourings, and in most food especially the highly refined and pre-packed foods. Even many imported fresh fruits are automatically sprayed with preservatives before shipment (to get rid of these, the fruit should be placed in hot water before it is eaten).

Most people do not realise or appreciate how detrimental this huge intake of chemicals is to their systems and to their own health. Only a few years ago, it was said that the American nation had turned into nutritional illiterates, and that it was an irresponsible act that the development of fabricated foods contained nothing but calories. How true those words turned out to be, but no more, for there is now becoming a new outlook on nutrition as the millions of Ch'ang Ming eaters testify, through their awareness of the Tao, their understanding of the fundamental laws of the universe, and through this consciousness they now recognise that ill health is absolutely unnecessary, and it is the fault of the ignorant if they become sick, or have their children born mentally retarded, or have physical deformity as part of their heritage. In addition to this, there are now many more children being born under weight, because of the weight consciousness of the mother.

To be truly fit to eat, food should be organically grown, without the aid of pesticides or artificial fertilisers, and should be completely unprocessed, so that it retains its natural nutritional constituents. This is how food was in the time of your great-grandparents, and in their day there were fewer cases of serious disease, and cancer had not been heard about. So start eating natural wholesome foods, making your diet consist of whole grain foods including brown rice, and vegetables preferably locally grown, and you will be amazed at the changes that come over you in so many different ways, and all to your personal benefit.

Get into the habit of chewing every mouthful of food at least fifty times, and more if you can. Let every mouthful turn into water before you swallow, and not only will you taste and appreciate the true flavour of the food that you are eating, but you will save your bowel systems a great deal of work. By so doing, you will get less acidity in the stomach, and your intestines will not need to take so long to do their work. If however, you gulp your food, then it will remain in the system for long periods whilst it digests and rots, and this rotting process creates a lot of harmful bacteria. If you have ever smelt a dung heap that has been standing for a long time, you will appreciate what your guts are like when the food has lain there a long while.

Never eat too much, and don't let your eyes be bigger than your belly; for this is a sure way of upsetting your system by over-loading it. If you eat moderately this will show through in personal forbearance and attitudes, and this change in disposition will lay the foundation for continual emotional equilibrium.

Reducing your liquid intake is also not an easy thing to do, because everything you eat contains fluid. Vegetables, for instance, are about 80 per cent water; rice is about 70 per cent water; and even toast has about 10 per cent moisture in it. When you consider that your body also consists of about 75 per cent fluid, it is obvious that a large intake of fluid is completely unnecessary.

Too much liquid will swell the tissues in the kidneys to such a degree that they will not be able to filter properly; this in turn will reduce or stop the amount of fluid that can pass through; and so the kidneys will become blocked. To help your kidneys, DRINK LESS of the obvious liquids such as teas, soups, fruit drinks etc., and your health will certainly benefit.

If at any time your mouth or the back of your throat feels dry, just adopt this Taoist habit, put the tongue against the roof of your mouth and in a few seconds you will find that your mouth fills up with saliva, which, when swallowed gently, will ease the dryness. If you get into this Taoist habit of keeping your tongue in this position, you will never feel dry and thirsty, and again, your health will receive the benefit.

The average person uses only two-thirds of his lung capacity each day, and by so doing, this helps to create the risk of lung troubles, headaches, worry, tension, insomnia, constipation and swelling round the stomach, and as oxygen is vital to the continual purification of the blood, you will appreciate the importance of correct breathing.

In the Taoist arts we have many specialised breathing exercises (basically, eight Yin breaths, eight Yang breaths, and four Yin-Yang); but there are also many more, some of which are used in healing, others to activate the Ch'i and others to promote good health. However, you do not have to be so particular, just get into the habit of breathing deeply through the nose at all times. This will relax the system, reduce tension, and encourage deep sleep.

A good barometer of the health is how long you need to sleep. If you are truly healthy, four to six hours each night should be enough for you to have all the vitality you need; you should also be able to wake up at any pre-determined time that you want, without using an alarm clock; and you should be able to fall asleep within thirty seconds, at any time of the day or night, and in any position. If you dream, snore or talk in your sleep, then you are unhealthy.

Food is the natural life-line of the human body and by eating the correct foods, suitable to the environment that we live in, we can ensure that the health of our anatomy can remain constantly good, and that we can maintain the vitality and energy within it, so that it will be strong enough to fight off all bacteria that might try and break through its natural defence system.

Not only can Ch'ang Ming help to keep everyone in good health all the time, but it will help the very thin person to put on weight, and the fat person to slim without the necessity of starving themselves or counting the calories. It can combat disease and also heal the sick and suffering, by the simple process of making the body strong enough to cure itself. After all, the Supreme Spirit made the human body in such a way that it should be able to repair itself continuously, and Ch'ang Ming is a way of making sure that the body does the job as efficiently as it was made to do, no matter whether the person is young or old.

Even the most serious complaints can be beaten and subdued, so that the person involved can be brought to a stage of permanent good health. Unfortunately there is one proviso—the body must not have been allowed to depreciate or to have deteriorated to such a low degree that it can no longer be aided to fight back in the space of time available—but there is always hope. In other words, it is like the house that was left to rot, it has almost become a pile of useless rubble. Two of the worst means to attain a useless and worthless body is to take drugs and to have unnecessary operations, both of these are only used in China when all other methods have failed, or in the case of broken bones and fractures etc. The warning is plain, if you are ill, or suffering from any complaint whatsoever, change to a Ch'ang Ming diet straight away and seek advice from the nearest Brocade Advisory Centre.

In the first ten days after starting a Ch'ang Ming health diet, you will begin to notice slight changes and certainly start to feel much better. However, between about ten days and a month of starting the diet, there may, in a few cases, be a few symptoms of change that may cause you to worry.

For instance, you may suffer diarrhoea or constipation. The diarrhoea signifies that the body is ridding itself of water, fat, carbohydrate, sugar and excess protein, and through this discharge you will lose weight even though you are eating well. This is nothing to worry about, for the body is making a natural adjustment, and it will eventually settle down to its natural weight level for its size.

Constipation may occur where the former diet included a large amount of fluid, and the condition may persist for two or three weeks. What happens is that, when there is a large intake of fluid the intestines become expanded and loose, and getting rid of the fluid causes the intestines to contract (rather like a balloon going down). As a result, peristalsis (the rippling effect of the muscular tissue of the intestines that passes the motion along to the anus) does not occur, and therefore constipation results. However, whereas constipation normally causes the mind to become a little slow and dull, it is not so in this case, and the mind becomes clear, and even sharp, because of the clearance of the waste and toxins.

If, during the first month of a Ch'ang Ming diet, you feel some aches or pains, make a note of them, for these show the various weaknesses that were in your body but which were hidden from you by the toxins. Once these toxins are drawn away there are contractions of the tissues and this creates a little tension, but the tension soon disappears and the aches and pains go with it.

In rare cases, women may find that their menstruations seem to go haywire and even stop for some months. Again, however, it is a case of the body healing the weaknesses first, and this may take some time. Once the weaknesses in the organs have been repaired, those in the bowel systems will be tackled, then those in the tissues, and then the sexual organs. As this process, of healing all the way through, is a slow procedure, it may take time to cure and heal every part of the body, especially if there happen to be many weaknesses—but remember, all these signs are an indication to you that the body is doing its dynamic work of healing within itself.

Grains (Wuku)
Always eat natural, unrefined whole grain such as brown rice, barley, buckwheat, millet, oats, wheat, rye, maize, but you should always make sure that you chew all grain food really well, as it contains fibre, which takes a lot of digesting, and you should help it to pass through the system as easily as possible. It also contains a lot of nutrition, and that is why it is excellent for the body, and it can be eaten in a variety of different ways—raw, creamed, fried, boiled and even baked so that there can be variety at every meal.

Brown rice is excellent for the nervous system; barley has a high energy level and is good for people suffering from various allergies; buckwheat is rich in Vitamin E, which is excellent for strengthening the tissues of the body and is beneficial to the kidneys; maize is another energy cereal and it is excellent for the blood; millet, on the other hand, is very beneficial to the spleen and especially for those people who suffer from acidosis; oats also have a high energy level, and are very good for people who have thyroid-gland troubles; rye is good for the tissues and muscular systems, and aids the endurance of those who perform strenuous activities; and wheat has long been known as an excellent tonic for the brain, is high in protein and gluten and is beneficial to the liver. So eat grain as often as you can, for it will give you excellent nourishment and will provide you with more than a quarter of the energy and nutrients that your body requires.

Here are a few ideas on how to prepare grain foods for the table.

Rice milk (Mi Nai).
All grains can be turned into a milk, but rice milk is really excellent for babies, the old, those people who have weak constitutions, and those with intestinal troubles.

Cook one cup of brown rice with ten cups of water for at least two hours, ensuring that you stir it continuously. Then place in a cloth and squeeze out all the juice. Boil the rice water again for fifteen minutes or longer, if you wish. For babies and people who are very weak the rice milk can be diluted to a weaker consistency, but for healthy folk they can have it stronger, by using less water. The rice pulp can be used when making bread. The same procedure holds good for the preparation of other grain milks too.

Millet cream (Hsiaomi Yu)
Warm one teaspoon of corn oil (or sesame or sunflower oil); add one cup of millet flour and stir until the mixture is a light brown; then let it cool. Put it into a pan and add four cups of water; boil; then allow it to simmer for fifteen to twenty minutes, stirring occasionally. Add a little soya sauce or sea salt to taste. Other grains may be used in place of millet.

Buckwheat herb (Ch'iaomai Ts'ao)
Cook the buckwheat in water and make a sauce from two dessertspoonfuls of any grain flour; then add some herbs, which should be chopped finely. Add the buckwheat, some steamed or baked onions and add a little oil; then cook until the grains are soft. Serve. Other grains may be used in place of the buckwheat.

Sauté buckwheat (Ch'ao Ch'iaomai)
Follow the instructions as for the buckwheat herb, then add garlic and marjoram, cut into the shape required, and sauté on both sides until they are a nice golden brown.

Vegetables (Ts'ai)
Vegetables, by which is meant not only the cultivated ones, but also wild ones such as dandelion, burdock and watercress, etc. which most people accept as herbs, are excellent for the bloodstream for they assist in the health of the red globules which carry the oxygen throughout the body. Vegetables can also supply appreciable quantities of various nutrients, including Vitamin C; but if the vegetables are allowed to wilt then there is considerable loss of this vitamin. So always ensure that you use fresh vegetables whenever you can, and, to obtain the maximum benefit from them, eat them raw or sauté them as we do in China.

Soya beans (Ta Tou)
The most valuable of vegetables is the soya bean, for it is a source

of dynamic goodness and excellent nutrition, and it is not for nothing that the Chinese have cultivated it for thousands of years. It is the only vegetable that contains complete nourishment and protein, such as Vitamins A, B, E, plenty of Vitamin C, and copper, iron, calcium, magnesium, nitrogen, zinc, phosphorous, potassium, sulphur, and in addition to all these it is very rich in lecithin.

Lecithin is essential for the tissues of the nervous system and the brain, as it aids the development of internal energy, and it is therefore important to help strengthen the nervous energy within the body. In addition to all this, it helps to break up excess fat in the body, so it is an excellent food for all those people who are carrying too much weight.

At home you can easily grow soya beans in a bottle in a few days, and they can either be used as a cooked vegetable, or eaten raw as part of a salad.

Soya bean flour (Ta Tou Fen)

It might surprise you to know that you can get Soya bean flour, and it can be used in bread, cakes, biscuits, and it makes them very tasty, and it can also be used to mix with other flours, where an added flavour is required. It can also be added to soups and gravies for the same reason.

In addition to the soya bean being used as nutritional flour, here are a few more of its uses either as a food or a drink.

Soya sauce (Chiangyu)

This is a fermented preparation from soya beans, and has been in China for at least 4,000–5,000 years. It adds to the flavour of food if used in reasonable quantities, and whilst it is rich in vitamins and minerals it also contains about 18 per cent salt.

Soya bean sweet (Ta Tou T'ang)

Boil the soya beans in syrup, drain, and then serve as a sweet.

Roasted soya beans (Ta Tou Ch'ao)

Soak the soya beans overnight, then roast them in a dry pan.

Roasted soya bean sweets (Ta Tou Ch'ao T'ang)

Roast the beans, then boil them in syrup, drain and serve.

Soya sauce pickled vegetables (Chiang Ts'ai)
Pickling vegetables in soya sauce not only gives them a wonderful flavour but gives them further nourishment.

Soya bean milk (Ta Tou Nai)
This has been used in China for thousands of years, and would always be used in preference to cows' milk, even to feed the young babies. You can make it yourself, by the same method as grain milk, or you can buy it in powder form. It is cheaper than other milk, and your health shop may already stock it. Go and ask.

Soya bean curd (Ta Tou Fu or Tou Fu)
This is one of the very old traditional foods of China and is also rich in protein. It can be used raw or added to soups and gravies and other dishes. This is the way you can make it yourself.

You will need half to one pound of soya beans, a little milk, some yeast, and sea salt to taste. Cook the beans; then, when nearly done, drain off most of the water into a bottle and seal it so that it is air-tight. Continue cooking until the beans are tender, then empty them into an earthenware dish and leave over-night. Reheat the next day and drain off the rest of the fluid. Add this to the liquid you had drained off the previous day. Pass the beans through a fine mesh sieve; add the puree to the liquid; and add a little milk, and some of the yeast, to aid fermentation, and add a little salt to suit your own taste. Divide into the sizes that you prefer, and then allow it to set.

Soya bean curd is also used as a compress to relieve aches and pains and areas of the body that are inflamed.

Seaweed (Hai Tai)
Another excellent vegetable is edible seaweed, for not only does it contain many vitamins, but it is also the best source of iodine, which is essential to the health of the body, and should be a part of everyone's diet, as it is in China.

Poisonous vegetables
There are a number of vegetables that contain poison and so are best left alone. These are potatoes, tomatoes, aubergines (egg-plants), spinach and rhubarb which contain solanine or oxalic

poison and these are harmful to the nervous system, create apathy, reduce the efficiency of the mind, and have other ill effects. In China, herds of pigs were fed on potatoes, and after a while they became more upset and very aggressive, and finally many of them developed arthritis and gout, and many died. So all these are best left out of your diet, if you want to keep fit and healthy.

Meat (Jou)
The consumption of meat has more disadvantages then benefits. It can supply quick energy and a large amount of calories, but once it has been swallowed it starts to decompose through the action of bacteria (throw a piece of meat on the ground and watch what happens to it), and this in turn creates toxins in the system. If the body cannot eliminate these quickly enough, the toxins have to be stored within the body, and this can cause fevers and many illnesses of the organs and the blood including blood stagnation.

Taoists do not eat red flesh, the reason being that thousands of years ago they went through a period when they ate only meat, in their quest for physical alchemy. They learnt dearly then, and appreciated the devastating effect and cost was to human lives—namely themselves, and they will never put themselves in that situation ever again.

When man first roamed the earth he had no weapons, and he had to live quite naturally on grains, vegetables and fruit; and he was at peace with the rest of the animal kingdom. When he began killing for flesh to eat, and wearing skins, animals and birds instinctively began to shy away from him, for their instincts told them that man was no longer a friend of nature, for he had become a killer. Since then, time has proved how right the animal world was, for man not only kills for food, but kills for pleasure, kills other humans, and in some cases kills himself by committing suicide—all of which can be seen as a state of degeneration.

The red flesh of man is exactly the same as the red flesh of animals, so man has turned into a cannibal by eating flesh, and whereas animals do not think and survival comes only through their inborn instincts, man does not have the same excuse, for he is slowly losing his capacity to think clearly and to use his judgement sensibly.

If he carries on at this rate of deterioration then he will eventually become lower than the animals he despises and hunts, then he will become the hunted and not the hunter. When will man understand that if you lower yourself down to the level of an animal then you will eventually become one yourself. Just look at local governments, for instance, every day they sit and make new laws, purposely to restrict and harness their fellow men, no animal does that, for it is an inborn instinct to seek continuous freedom, and not perpetual shackles.

Therefore if everyone raised their standard of eating and drinking according to the divine laws of the universe, then they will eventually raise themselves to the heights of the teachers, philosophers and sages, and become an example to all their fellow men. Then will come peace, happiness and harmony amongst all humanity, and war, robbery, mugging, and rape will be things of the past.

Milk (Nai)

We have already noticed the old Chinese saying, "If you want your child to grow up to look and act like an animal, then feed it on cows' or goats' milk from the day it is born". For this reason, the Chinese generally do not feed animal milk to their babies, and it is not unknown for Chinese mothers to breast-feed their children for as much as three to five years. Children fed this way tend to have a more adaptable mind, more flexibility in the body and a calmer and stronger spirit.

It is simply not true that cows' milk is the complete food for man, for it is deficient in iron and Vitamin C and D, and if bottled milk is left on the doorstep exposed to the sunlight for an hour or more, a substantial amount of its Vitamin C and riboflavin is destroyed. Cows' milk also contains an appreciable quantity of carbohydrate, in the form of disaccharide lactose.

In Great Britain most milk is pasteurised and this treatment destroys about 10 per cent of thiamine and Vitamin B and about 25 per cent of Vitamin C. In sterilised and evaporated milk the losses are much higher amounting to 60 per cent of Vitamin C and 20 per cent of thiamine. In some countries they even add chemicals in the form of preservatives to milk, and these too destroy some of the vital nutrients.

So it is well worth remembering that: *COWS' MILK WAS*

MADE FOR CALVES, HUMAN MILK WAS MADE FOR HUMAN BABIES. You wouldn't feed human milk to animals, so why feed animal milk to humans? Everything in nature has its rightful place, so let it stay that way, as the Supreme Spirit intended it to be.

Salt (Yen)

Ordinary rock salt does more harm than good to the human body, for it causes the retention of too much fluid, which in turn can cause the body to put on surplus weight and it can lead to heart trouble, high blood pressure, ulcers, fatigue, insomnia as well as a violent and aggressive nature. It contains very little goodness, as most of that evaporated in the far distant past; so today its main constituent is sodium chloride.

Sea salt (Tsao Yen), which contains many minerals from the sea, is far more beneficial to the human body, but it should be used in moderation. However, in China we find it an even greater advantage to the natural good health of the body, to use salt in other forms, such as Soya sauce (Chiangyu) and Sesame seed salt (Chihma Yen), and these help to make the food more tasty and supply sea salt in a way that it is more acceptable to the human body, but remember—moderation at all times.

Chapter 11

Herbs for Health

The importance of herbs has been acknowledged by people of all nations, but the Chinese, through the infinite wisdom of the "Sons of Reflected Light", were given a wonderful start at understanding the value and properties of them.

At around 3,000 BC, Shen Nung, later known as Huang Ti (the Yellow Emperor), drew up a list of hundreds of herbs and specified their useful and harmful properties After his death he was given the title of "The Divine Husbandman" (he is also credited with the invention of the plough and construction of the first wheeled cart, with devising various systems of irrigation, and with extending the arts of husbandry) and was chosen to be one of the gods of the apothecaries of China. He is probably best known for his classic of Chinese internal medicine, the *Nei Ching*, which to this day is widely consulted by physicians.

Since the reign of the Yellow Emperor the tremendous work of listing all the herbs and their properties has continued, and today Chinese traditional medicine recognises over 30,000 herbs and has at its disposal even more recipes for the use of them. The herbs are of course, subject to the Yin and Yang influences, as is everything else in the universe, and they can be used internally or externally or both at once. Their efficacy has been proved over thousands of years, but depends on the proper use of them (i.e. when and how they are taken or administered).

When being used internally, they can, for instance, be taken hot or cold, in the form of pills, powders, drinks or soups, depending on need. For certain complaints they may need to be administered before a meal; for others after; sometimes in the very early morning, on an empty stomach; and sometimes in the late evening after the last meal has been digested. According to the illness, a slow, gentle influence, working over a long period, may be required, or the need may be for a quick expansion, with rapid results.

Similar considerations apply to external use. Should the preparation be applied hot or cold, over a long period or a short period? How much of the body should it cover? Does it need to penetrate the body only a little way, or must it have a very deep effect?

Whilst the internal is Yin and the external is Yang, everything, as we have seen earlier, has something of both, and a balance needs to be maintained. That is why people living in the colder climates (Yin) should eat more Yang foods, whilst those living in the tropics (Yang) should concentrate on more Yin foods (always remembering that the food in question should be naturally and locally grown, and that nothing should be consumed in excess).

The ancient herbal textbooks classify the whole range of herbs into five categories:

1. those that are nutritious and can be mixed with the food of a Ch'ang Ming diet;
2. those herbs that can be used in medicines and are non-poisonous;
3. poisonous herbs that may be used in very small quantities;
4. herbs which can be used only for a short period of time; and
5. herbs that can be safely used over long periods.

Most of the herbs that grow in the West are also known and found in China, but the size and climatic variety of China is such that many herbs that are found there do not occur in the West. In this chapter we shall concentrate on herbs that can be grown or are readily purchasable in the West, and shall pay particular regard to their health-giving properties. Shortage of space means that only a selection of herbs can be covered.

Onions (Ts'ung)

These are rich in Vitamin C and are excellent for the kidneys, but in their raw state they should be consumed only in small quantities. They are very good for those who suffer from flatulence, diabetes, hardening of the arteries, colds, influenza or asthma, they help to increase the appetite, and they encourage sleep.

Onion drink (Ts'ung K'ou). A nasal discharge, a cold or asthma can be eradicated simply by dipping a slice of raw onion into a glass of hot water for a few seconds, then sipping the water slowly throughout the day. This drink will also stimulate the kidneys.

Onion gruel (Ts'ung Chou). Boil the onions in water, and, having removed the onions, use the water to make a gruel from brown rice, oats or other grains. This, consumed in the evening, will be found to induce sleep.

Onion poultice (Ts'ung Pa). This is prepared from onions chopped finely and placed between two cloths, and if applied to the neck will quickly disperse colds, headaches and even earache. When applied to the kidneys it will help stimulate them, and if applied to the calves of the legs will relieve heart trouble. If the onions are heated before being placed between the cloths, the poultice will greatly aid the circulation in the area to which it is applied, and so is good for gout, arthritis and stomach pains.

Radishes (Lo Po)

Radishes are an excellent remedy for liver disorders, but an excess can prove harmful. A teaspoonful of neat raw radish juice is the largest dose permitted in one day.

Radish tea (Lo Po Ch'a). Dried grated radishes or a small amount of radish juice should be added to water and allowed to simmer in a pan for about five minutes. If you have used dried radishes, strain the liquid before serving. This is good for the kidneys and will aid the passing of urine where there is urine retention.

Radish syrup tea (Lo Po T'ang Chiang Ch'a). Prepare as radish tea, using radish syrup.

Radish syrup (Lo Po T'ang Chiang). Squeeze the juice out of some grated radishes, then put the juice into a pan over a low flame. Add honey, molasses or sugar, but only enough to turn the juice into a thick syrup. If you bottle it in an air-tight container it will keep for some time. Radish syrup is excellent against gall-stones, whooping cough and bronchial catarrh. For gall stones, a quarter teaspoonful in a tablespoonful of water should be taken three times a day. For coughs and catarrh, add a quarter teaspoonful to half a cup of water, which should be sipped slowly throughout the day.

Radish juice (Lo Po Chih). Grate the radish and squeeze one cup of juice from it, then put it into a pan together with one cup of water. Heat, and remove as soon as it boils. Radish juice is very good for the kidneys, aids urination, and is effective against skin troubles (e.g. ulcers, boils and other swellings). Take a cupful once a day for two days, then wait a few days, and, if the condition still persists, repeat.

Ginger radish (Chiang Lo Po). Boil one pint of water, then add three tablespoonfuls of grated radish, a half teaspoonful of grated ginger or ginger powder, and one teaspoonful of soya sauce. This is wonderfully effective against liver troubles, and by inducing sweating can reduce fevers. Drink a wineglassful in the evening.

Garlic (Suan)

Though disliked by many because of its pungent smell, garlic has many excellent qualities. It can be used as a stimulant, a diuretic, an expectorant, an anti-spasmodic, and a strong rubefacient, for when applied directly to the skin it causes a nasty blister. It can be added to food or used as a medicine. It is effective against intestinal malfunctions of all kinds (indigestion, worms, flatulence, and so on), respiratory infections (coughs, whooping cough, asthma, bronchitis, catarrh), and hypertension (high blood pressure). In places where it is used as part of the daily diet, cancer is virtually unknown. It assists the body to retain youthfulness and sexual vigour; it is good against all skin complaints and will quickly heal open sores, scratches and wounds; and it enters the bloodstream and so circulates the entire body, eradicating harmful bacteria, expelling toxins, and benefiting the tissues and membranes.

Garlic oil (Suan Yu) Because of garlic's rubefacient qualities, it is in many cases much better to use the oil than the clove, especially when giving it to young children and old people. This oil is readily purchasable (usually in the form of "pearles") from health shops and herbalists.

Garlic milk (Suan Nai) is really excellent for the treatment of intestinal disorders, sciatica, rheumatism and arthritis, and it can also be successfully used as an enema. Stir two grated or crushed cloves of garlic into a quarter-pint of warm milk, and drink. Garlic oil may be used in place of cloves. Normally the preparation should be taken at least twice a day, night and morning.

Garlic bread (Suan Mienpao). For this use about three cloves of garlic (or the equivalent garlic oil) to one pound of flour, baking in the normal way. This is very tasty and an excellent way of taking the garlic.

Garlic poultice (Suan Kaoyao). Crush or finely chop the cloves of garlic; spread evenly over a soft cloth to a depth of about a quarter of an inch; then place another cloth over the top of the garlic. (Remember that garlic will burn and blister the skin if brought directly into contact with it.) The poultice is excellent against scabies, boils, abscesses and other skin complaints. If the garlic is heated in a frying pan and put into a compress, it is very good against breast cancer.

For whooping coughs, bronchial or other hacking coughs, apply garlic poultices to the soles of the feet, then wear old socks over the top to hold the poultices in place during the night. You can use the same compress over and over again.

Ginseng (Jenshen)

A complete book could be written about this herb, which has been used in China for well over 5,000 years, and a number of mythological tales have been built around it and its healing qualities, which are manifold. It can cure or relieve very many complaints.

As a pep to the energy level of the body it is excellent, and it will revitalise the mentally tired and the physically run down. It will eradicate the effects of a hangover after a good night out, will soothe an inflamed stomach, and will overcome digestive upsets, including flatulence and heartburn. It is a wonderful tranquilliser, relieving nervous disorders, depression, fainting, drowsiness, and headaches, and quickly cures respiratory conditions such as coughs, asthma and sinus trouble. When mixed with comfrey it will stop the most obstinate internal bleeding through the mouth, nose or anus.

Ginseng tea (Jenshen Ch'a). Add one ounce of ginseng to two cups of water, and boil until about the quantity of one cupful. This is the dosage for stomach upsets and nervous complaints. If possible, should be taken morning, noon and night.

Ginseng nuts (Jenshen Ho-erh). Take an ounce of ginseng powder, mix it with a little honey, and roll into balls about the size of the nail of the little finger. Place one of them under the tongue of the mouth. When it has completely dissolved replace with another. This will stop coughs very quickly, and will also help to dissolve any excess phlegm in the throat.

Ginseng milk (Jenshen Nai). Boil one ounce of ginseng in a cup and a half of water until it reduces to about three-quarters of a cupful; then mix with two cups of rice milk. Honey can be added if desired. Ginseng milk is very good for old people whose energy is failing or who are feeling very weak; and it is excellent for frail children and people with a weak sexual drive. It is also a great help in the fight against cancer, and will help accelerate the cure of it.

Ginseng essence (Jenshen Ch'ing). Boil one ounce of ginseng in one cup of water until only the sediment is left. Store in an air-tight glass or earthenware container until required. This essence can be added to soups, medications and flour, for added goodness.

Ginseng and orange peel (Jenshen Ch'enp'i). Mix equal parts of ginseng and dried, powdered orange peel in a little hot water. After the mixture has cooled slightly, add an ample amount of honey. Drink this just before going to bed, in order to counteract insomnia and restlessness.

Parsley (Hsiang Ts'ai)

Parsley tends these days to be relegated to a decoration for food, when really it contains more goodness than a lot of the food that it is used to decorate. It is very rich in Vitamin A, has more Vitamin C than oranges, and greatly stimulates the bladder and the kidneys, so helping to dispel stones and gravel and cure disorders of these organs. In China it used to counteract malaria, jaundice and dropsy. The whole of the plant is used, but in the West it is mainly the leaves and seeds that are used.

Parsley tea (Hsiang Ts'ai Ch'a). Add half a cup of firmly packed parsley leaves, or leaves and stems, to one pint of boiling water and allow to soak for fifteen minutes. Strain and bottle in an air-tight container, and cool quickly. Have a wineglassful daily and add a drop of soya sauce to each.

Sage (Sheng Jen)

Sage has always played an important part in salads, stuffings, and sauces and has been used over the centuries for adding flavour to cheese. If you make your own cottage or vegetarian cheese add this wonderful herb to give it that bit more taste and goodness. In China it is sometimes added to soya-bean cheese and curd. Sage is excellent in treating weak appetities, nervous ailments, upset livers and kidney troubles, and it helps ensure that menstruation is regular. However, nursing mothers should not drink sage tea, as it has a tendency to stop the milk in the breasts.

Sage tea (Sheng Jen Ch'a). Add half an ounce of sage leaves and stems to one pint of hot water. (Do not boil the water, as otherwise you will lose the benefit of the volatile oil that the sage contains.) Drink a wineglassful daily.

Sage gargle (Sheng Jen Shuk'ou). Mix one ounce of sage with two ounces of honey and one dram of borax; steep the mixture in one pint of hot (not boiling) water for fifteen to twenty minutes; allow to cool, then strain and bottle. For a sore or inflamed throat, laryngitis, tonsilitis or mouth ulcers, use the gargle three times daily.

Mint (Po-he).

Every housewife or herbalist uses mint at some time or another. It is added to food and used in teas, soups, soft drinks, sauces, wines, sweets and even bath preparations (in some cases it is the oil and acids extracted from the leaves that are used). It is soothing and cooling to the system and very beneficial to the digestive organs, for it eases flatulence and helps to increase the appetite. It expels internal fevers, activates perspiration and reduces swellings.

For medicinal purposes the whole plant is used. Mint tea (Po-he Ch'a) can be drunk three or four times daily, or can be used externally for bathing inflamed parts of the body.

Fennel (Hui Hsiang)

Fennel is very easy to grow in the garden and is not only aromatic but also, owing to its yellow flowers, very pretty. In the West, fennel is mainly used to enhance fish dishes, but it can also be used as a constituent of salads. For this, peel and chop a little of the stems, which you should cut before the flowers appear (in autumn).

Fennel is a sweet-tasting herb and an excellent tonic; it helps the digestive system, disperses flatulence, breaks up phlegm, helps to get rid of surplus fat, and stimulates milk production in mothers. For those suffering from gastro-enteritis, hernia, severe intestinal pains, liver disorders or jaundice, it is a *must*.

Fennel tea (Hui Hsiang Ch'a). Use a quarter of an ounce of fennel seeds to one pint of boiling water, and sip during the day.

Burdock (Niu P'ang Tzu)

Burdock grows in profusion almost anywhere, especially in

damp places. The seeds, leaves and the roots are all used in Chinese herbal therapy, while the stalks, stripped of their tough outer skin, are used as a vegetable in salads and other dishes. Burdock helps the bladder and the kidneys to function efficiently, cures influenza and tonsilitis, clears fevers, disperses wind, aids damaged tissues to heal rapidly, speeds up perspiration when needed, and is effective against many skin troubles, such as boils and abscesses.

Burdock tea (Niu P'ang Tzu Ch'a). Add a quarter-ounce of burdock seeds to one pint of boiling water. Drink one wineglassful three times daily.

Burdock poultice (Niu P'ang Tzu Pa). For external applications the roots and the leaves are crushed, warmed up and placed in a thin cloth, then applied to the part affected. This is effective against all skin troubles.

Tarragon (Ch'ing Hao)

This herb is generally thought of as one that has been cultivated only in Europe, but in fact it emanates originally from China. It is used to enhance fowl dishes and is commonly used in vinegar, pickles and tartare sauce. It is excellent when sprinkled over salads, but, being strongly aromatic, it should not be used with other herbs. It is beneficial to the heart, the liver, and the brain and strengthens the memory.

Tarragon tea (Ch'ing Hao Ch'a). If the leaves are dried, they lose some of their oil and flavour, so it is better to use fresh leaves. Use a quarter-ounce to one pint of hot water (dilute further if you find it too strong) and sip it slowly during the day. Dried tarragon is stocked by most herbalists and health shops, but the plant is very easy to grow.

Plantain (Che Ch'ien Tze)

This plant is very common, and is a well-known folk remedy for nettle and insect stings (the leaves are rubbed against the spot affected). In China, plantain is eaten as a spring green while the leaves are still young and tender and before the seed spikes begin to show. It is a beneficial salad vegetable, though slightly bitter. Plantain is a diuretic, soothes coughs, relieves diarrhoea and piles, is valuable in preventing excessive blood-clotting, and is said to increase sperm-production in man and fertility in woman.

Seaweed (Hai Tai)

Seaweed has been eaten in China for thousands of years, for it is very rich in vitamins and minerals. It contains iodine, Vitamins A, B and E, and traces of magnesium, copper, silver, titanium, nickel, chromium, barium, sulphur, sodium and many other minerals. It is eaten as a vegetable, and in powdered form is used as a condiment in place of salt and to add flavour and goodness to bread, biscuits, cakes and so forth. Seaweed prevents goitre, relieves congestion, breaks up phlegm, reduces fever, relieves heart trouble, brings down high blood pressure, and cures tumours, cysts and dropsy.

Seaweed tea (Hai Tai Ch'a). To one pint of boiling water add a quarter-ounce of seaweed or seaweed powder, and drink a wineglassful at each meal.

Seaweed compress (Hai Tai Kaoyao). Add two ounces of chopped seaweed to one pint of boiling water; dip a cloth into the fluid; squeeze it out; then apply to the painful joints.

Dandelion (P'u Kung Ying)

Though in many countries it is considered a weed, in China and France the dandelion is cultivated, on account of its nutritious tender leaves and excellent medicinal value. It is rich in Vitamins A and C, it contains more iron than spinach, and it has many other valuable constituents, including potassium. The tender young leaves, though slightly bitter, make a pleasant addition to salads, and they can be sautéed and mixed with soups. Excellent for the liver, heart, kidneys, stomach and bladder, dandelion is normally extremely fast-working, especially when taken in the form of tea.

Wonderful for the relief of digestive troubles, such as heartburn and wind, it quickly clears skin complaints, prevents gravel, assists in dissolving the alkaline deposits characteristic of gout and rheumatoid arthritis, disperses toxins and fevers, and may be used in the treatment of venereal diseases.

Dandelion tea (P'u Kung Ying Ch'a). Boil two ounces of chopped root or leaves, or a mixture of both, in two pints of water, and let it simmer until only one pint of liquid remains. Drink a small wineglassful every three hours.

Dandelion coffee (P'u Kung Ying K'afei). Take the roots only of a two-year-old plant; wash them, and dry them with a cloth; roast them in an oven until they are light brown; grind them; and store the powder in an air-tight container, where it will keep for months. It is an excellent substitute for real coffee, may be drunk by children as well as adults, and is an excellent bedtime drink, helping the body to relax and sleep deeply.

Rue (Yun Hsiang)

This beautiful little shrub is known in many parts of the world and can be bought dried from most health shops. In China the leaves and the roots are used in medication; but in other countries only the leaves or new shoots are used. Though the leaves have a slightly bitter taste and an aromatic smell, a little rue, chopped finely, is a good addition to a salad. Rue contains rutin, which is excellent for the circulation, but it should be taken only in very small doses. Rue also acts as a stimulant and tonic to the uterus, relieves congestion, fights colic and worms, and is considered to be a disinfectant protecting the body from virus infections and the like.

Rue tea (Yun Hsiang Ch'a). Add an ounce of rue to a pint of boiling water. Take in doses of a wineglassful every two or three hours, adding, if preferred, a little honey or soya sauce. This will ease excessive menstruation, coughs, colds, influenza, meningitis, sore throats, piles and hepatitis; will relieve aches and sprains, and the pains of rheumatoid arthritis; and will improve the eyesight of the aged.

Mugwort (Ai Yen)

Mugwort has long been used throughout China for both internal and external purposes, and it is still used there extensively. It should be used only in small doses, and, whilst it has a bitter taste, it is fragrant and warming. It stops bleeding (including hæmatemesis), stimulates the appetite, helps rectify irregular menstruation, is effective against skin complaints, restores energy levels, and dispels wind and abdominal cramps.

Mugwort tea (Ai Yen Ch'a). Add one teaspoonful of mugwort to one pint of boiling water. Drink a wineglassful in the morning and in the evening.

Dates (Ts'ao)

Slowly simmer (flesh and stone together) in hot water until a thick liquid is obtained, drain off the sediment, and drink the water in doses of a dessertspoonful at a time. This is effective against weaknesses of the stomach and spleen, fatigue, low energy levels and anaemia; it soothes the heart and the lungs; and, for anyone whose mouth is continually dry, it activates the saliva.

Cinnamon (Joukui)

China has always been a big producer of this spice, which is also used in perfume sticks and joss sticks. Whilst it is pleasant to the taste, it is hot, and thus is good for warming the circulation, the kidneys, the heart and the abdomen. If you should catch a chill or a cold in the lungs, and are coughing and wheezing constantly, cinnamon will bring rapid relief.

Cinnamon tea (Joukui Ch'a) Mix a quarter-ounce of cinnamon powder in four cupfuls of water, and boil until only half the liquid remains. Take a small wineglassful before each meal (three times daily).

Licorice (Kan Ts'ao)

Added to various herb teas, licorice not only acts as a sweetener and renders harsher flavours more pleasant, but also may convert a Yin influence to a Yang one. Wonderful for the liver and the stomach, it is a very soothing laxative for old and young, soothes coughs and inflamed throats, and eases stomach and intestinal cramps and severe constipation. In China, it is also used to combat irregular menstruation, infertility in women, tuberculosis, pneumonia and pleurisy. The root is used in China in its natural state, but in the West it is advisable to buy the licorice sticks (made from the juice of the root after it has been crushed and boiled) sold by herbalists and health shops.

As it absorbs water, anyone who is over-weight should not include licorice in their diet; but, in the case of those who are thin or dehydrated, licorice will help the body retain fluid.

Dosage (Fu). Add one three-inch stick of licorice to half a pint of hot water and allow to dissolve; if you prefer, add a little honey or soya sauce. Drink a small wineglassful about thirty minutes before a meal.

Rhubarb (Ta Huang)

In China, rhubarb stalks are not eaten, because of the poison they contain, and the leaves are even more dangerous. However, the root has excellent medicinal virtues and most herbalists sell it, in powder form or otherwise. It is excellent for the treatment of constipation, diarrhoea, dysentery, fever, coughs, bad breath, colitis, dropsy and disease of the heart. It breaks down blood clots, boils and purulent ulcers. Being very Yin, it will help to expel heat in the case of jaundice.

Dosage (Fu). Mix a little hot water with a quarter-ounce of rhubarb root powder, adding a little honey if desired. Take early in the morning.

Rhubarb oil (Ta Huang Yu). This is extracted by squeezing the root. Take one teaspoonful before breakfast.

China tea (Chungkuo Ch'a)

Many types of tea are cultivated and made in China, but the two that are best from a medicinal point of view are the black tea and the green tea. They both help to fight colds, headaches, dysentry, and flatulence; aid the circulation; and are reputed to strengthen weak eyes.

The black tea from Fukien is a little difficult to acquire, as it is grown only in a small area and foreign demand much exceeds the exports, but it is a really excellent tea and very aromatic. The green tea, by contrast, can be purchased quite easily, as it is produced in many areas of China and sufficient is exported. The Chinese are very particular about ensuring that the leaves retain the maximum goodness, and for that reason they pick them only in the very early morning, before the sun rises, and whilst they are still moist with dew.

Roasted tea (Ch'ao Ch'a). Roast the green tea until it turns brown, then prepare in the normal way. If you have a painful or bloodshot eye, put a little of this tea (only lukewarm) into an eyeglass and bathe the eye with it, and you will find that it will bring relief.

Soya green tea (Chiangyu Lu Ch'a). Add two tablespoonfuls of soya sauce to a cup of hot green tea, and drink it after a meal. This is excellent for insomnia, fatigue, headaches and stomach-ache, and for anyone who is suffering from shock or from an injury.

Salt green tea (Yen Lu Ch'a). Add one level teaspoonful of sea salt to one cup of lukewarm tea. This is excellent for rinsing the nasal passages to aid the discharge of mucus.

Ginger green tea (Chiang Lu Ch'a). To a cup of hot green tea add a pinch of ginger powder and stir well before drinking. This is very good for those who feel cold internally; for stomach upsets; and as an aid to menstruation.

Hawthorn (Yeh Shancha)

Although the flowers are edible and can be sprinkled on to fruit salads, yoghurt and custards, it is the roots and fruits that are used medicinally, for they are astringent and warming. They aid digestion, stop diarrhoea and dysentery, stimulate the circulation of the blood, and ease menstrual and abdominal cramps.

Dosage (Fu). Mix a quarter-ounce of the pulped fruits and roots with a little hot water. Taken twice daily.

Hawthorn compress (Yeh Shancha Kaoyao). Put a little hot water with the pulped roots and fruit, and mix it with a little flour so that it attains a thick consistency. Apply to the painful area and hold in place with a cloth or bandage. If you place a hot-water bottle on top of the bandage, this will increase the time for which the heat is retained.

Charcoal (Mut'an)

Hyper-acidity of the stomach causes heartburn and results from an excess of Yin foods, especially meat and dairy produce. The toxins derived from these make gastric secretions.

A very ancient Chinese remedy for this condition is to mix one teaspoonful of charcoal powder with a cup of green tea, straining the sediment off before drinking it. Another recipe is to mix one teaspoonful of charcoal powder with rice milk or any other grain milk, making sure that you strain it before drinking. In either case, the acidity will be very quickly neutralised.

Sesame seeds (Chihma)

These little seeds contain an abundance of protein and minerals, including an ample supply of calcium, which, combined with their natural unsaturated oil, makes them an excellent food and one that is easily assimilated by the body. They are an excellent tonic for the liver and kidneys, and the oil is good for the organs of the body. They are used to combat constipation and skin complaints and to strengthen the nerves and heart muscles, and the oil helps supply the body with oxygen, which is essential in preventing cancer.

Sesame-seed tea (Chihma Ch'a). Mix a quarter-ounce of sesame seeds with two cupfuls of water and boil until only half the liquid remains; strain off the sediment and drink the fluid. Take before meals (three times daily).

Sesame-seed sauté (Chien Chihma). Warm a dry pan over a low flame; add your sesame seeds and continually stir them as they fry in their own oil. Once they are crisp, allow to cool and then store in an air-tight container. These seeds can be eaten at any time, and it is a good idea to carry some with you, to chew now and then; but make sure that you chew them really well.

Sesame-seed salt (Chihma Yen). Heat sesame seeds and then crush them gently in a mortar with a pestle; add sea salt (one part to five parts sesame seeds) and reheat; then crush until a coarse powder. Store in an air-tight container, and use as a condiment. (Most health shops now sell sesame-seed salt ready made.)

Sesame seed and ginger (Chihma Chiang). Mix one teaspoonful of sesame-seed oil with one teaspoonful of ginger juice or essence; warm only slightly; then apply to the scalp to combat dandruff and loss of hair.

Sesame-seed oil (Chihma Yu). Heat some sesame-seeds, then filter the oil through a piece of very fine cotton or muslin. Store in an air-tight glass container and allow to cool. Obtain an eyedrop and apply one drop to each eye just before you fall to sleep. It will sting or smart for the first night or two, but thereafter you will feel nothing. This is excellent for those with weak eyesight, and anyone suffering from any form of eye trouble. It is also very good for those people with good, strong eyes, as it helps the lubrication of the eyes and gives added protection.

If you have suffered a cut or abrasion, or have had any skin operation, smear the area thinly with sesame-seed oil, for it is very soothing to inflamed areas, helps the skin to heal much more quickly, and helps to eradicate any scars.

Black sesame seeds (Hei Chihma)

These are excellent for treating liver and kidney malfunctions, head colds, constipation, numbness or paralysis. Follow the same recipes as for ordinary sesame seeds.

Pearl barley (Imi)

Pleasant to the palate, it strengthens the spleen, helps relieve rheumatoid arthritis, combats diarrhoea, lung abscesses, lobar pneumonia and appendicitis, and, because it has a tendency to convert moisture within the body, is a great help to all those who have difficulty in urination.

Dosage (Fu). Mix a quarter-ounce of pearl barley with two cups of water; boil until half the liquid remains; drain off the sediment; and drink morning and evening. Soya sauce can be added to give more flavour.

Ginger (Chiang)

Ginger's warmth (Yang) makes it invaluable in combating ailments caused or created through internal or external cold (Yin). It is of great benefit to the stomach and spleen, eases abdominal pains in women, relieves paralysed limbs and painful joints, aids the digestive organs, cures colds, diarrhoea, poor menstruation and nausea, expels worms, and may be used both extensively internally and externally in the fight against cancer.

Ginger sweets (Chiang T'ang). Mix some ginger with honey and form into balls about the size of the nail of your little finger. Chew one ball before meals.

Ginger tea (Chiang Ch'a). Add half a teaspoonful of ginger powder to one pint of boiling water and boil for fifteen to twenty minutes. Add honey or soya sauce to taste.

Roasted ginger (Ch'ao Chiang). Ginger powder can be dry-fried, and, once it has become crispy and changed colour, it can be made into a tea (see previous recipe), or applied to bleeding open sores, to stop the bleeding.

Ginger oil (Chiang Yu). You can either purchase this ready prepared, or obtain it by squeezing ginger root. Put one drop in the mouth and swallow slowly. This will tend to break up the phlegm in the throat and will ease constipation. Swallow three or four drops a day.

Ginger compress (Chiang Kaoyao). Put four ounces of ginger powder into a small muslin bag and tie the top. Drop into four pints of boiling water, and boil for twenty minutes. Every now and then squeeze the bag with a wooden spoon, so that as much as possible of the ginger is extracted. Leave the bag in the water.

Take a cloth or napkin, dip it into the ginger water, and apply it to the painful area of the body. As it tends to cool off fairly quickly, dip it back into the water, squeeze out, and apply again. Repeat this every three or four minutes, applying the compress for a total of fifteen minutes.

Don't throw the water away, but use it over and over again; and when it has all gone make yourself a fresh lot. This can be used externally for cancer, stomach pains and cramps, appendicitis, piles, leprosy, rheumatism, arthritic joints, and sterility in women.

We have now examined a few of the many herbs that are available for the benefit of humanity. Make use of them whenever you can, but remember that there is no herb that can cure every illness and that every remedy requires time to work. If you have suffered from arthritis for twenty years, don't expect it to disappear over night: but if you are dedicated you can expect to make steady progress.

Remember that if you take one aspirin it will take the body six months to get rid of every particle of it. If you take one "trip" on LSD, then it will take three years to get it all out of the system, and the same applies to a cortisone injection.

Remember too that it takes approximately ten months to grow new nails, it takes two and a half to three years to grow one layer of skin tissue, and it takes ten years to revitalise the bones. So, whilst the body will do its work for you faithfully and constantly, without thanks or rewards, you have got to look after it every day of your life if you are not to let yourself in for long periods of illness.

It is entirely in you own hands to safeguard your health, so don't go out in the cold with just the flimsiest of clothes on; keep away from Yin foods; and, above all, change to a Ch'ang Ming diet straightaway and stick to it for the rest of your life, and you will never need to look back.

Remember that Ch'ang Ming is not a fad, for it came into being before there were such things as fads. It is an *art* proved over thousands and thousands of years. You too can join the millions of former pale faces who eat the Ch'ang Ming way and are now pink faces. Write to the Chinese Cultural Arts Association, which will be pleased to hear from you and advise you at any time.

Chapter 12

Lose Weight Through the Benefits of Nutrition

"I have had bad nerves, heartburn, wind, tummy upsets, headaches, and also spasmodic periods of diarrhoea for many years now, and I get depressed so easily, but my biggest worry is my weight. I've been on calorie diets, cut down my food to a bare minimum on occasions, and have even been on a fast, yet it is all in vain, for I still keep putting on more and more weight. Yet, these days I hardly eat a thing, but it still doesn't make the slightest difference for the scales tell me I am getting heavier and heavier. Can you help me, for I so desperately need to take off some of it, for I know that I am grossly over-weight."

This is a plea that was addressed to me by a lady in South Wales, who, like so many Westerners in like case, had simply got her priorities all mixed up. Her concern to lose weight had caused her ill health, which in turn had aggravated her weight problem. To relieve her ailments she was taking a mass of drugs, which did not help her at all but only made things worse.

The first thing, naturally, was to find out the actual cause of the illnesses that she had been suffering for so long. A pulse study, together with a close look at her face, confirmed that her condition was entirely due to inflammation of the stomach, obviously owing to very bad eating and drinking habits over a long period of time. I advised her to start on a strict Ch'ang Ming diet, using also a few herbs; and so battle commenced.

Now three years have gone by and all of her illnesses have completely disappeared, she looks the picture of good health, and her family life is very happy indeed. Her weight has been reduced by three stone (20 kilograms) and is now fairly steady throughout the year.

Most Westerners are under the impression that by eating grain foods they will automatically put on a lot of unnecessary fat and extra weight. To test this assumption, the Chinese Cultural Arts Association (Ch'ang Ming Section) asked its London group members to participate in a weight experiment. All agreed to have a go, and for the purpose were divided into two groups, with an equal number of men and women in both.

One section was put on a low-calorie diet, while the other section went on to a 100 per cent grain diet, for two months. In that time, curiously enough, the people who were eating only grain lost more weight than those on the low-calorie diet, so proving what the Chinese have known all along. Take a look at any Chinese that you happen to meet, and, unless he has changed to Western eating habits, you will see that he is not fat or over-weight, even though he seems to eat a lot of rice, consumes Chinese pastries, and eats a lot of fried food.

This can be explained very simply. His main dish is rice, which is grain; most of his exquisite pastries are made from grain, rice or egg, and are therefore very light; and he does not deep-fry his food, but uses the sauté method, or what is sometimes referred to as "stir frying".

The real cause of the obesity that is now so common among occidentals is their excessive consumption of sugar, meat and protein, fruit, dairy produce, food containing added chemicals, and deep-fried foods. There is also the detrimental effect of alcohol and spirits to be taken into account.

So how is it that people can lose weight by eating grain food? The answer is actually very simple: whole-grain foods contain fibre or "roughage", which cannot be digested at all. To make sure that it passes through the body as early as possible, each mouthful must be chewed at least fifty times, to break this fibre up into minute fragments and to ensure that there is ample saliva to oil its downward flow. Now, grain foods are quite "filling", but the part of them that is only fibre (i.e. excluding the nutrients they contain) is waste and is passed out of the system, so that it does not serve to put on weight. Another important consideration is that whole-grain food does not create bacteria within the stomach to the same extent as meat, for instance, does, and so less toxin is produced, which in turn makes less water, which produces less fat, so that you lose weight. A grain diet stops you from overloading your stomach, and yet ensures that you consume sufficient nutrients to satisfy the needs of the body and keep it healthy.

If you are over-weight, the first thing to find out is by how much. To calculate the correct weight for your height, follow the simple method of calculation outlined in Chapter 6 above (under "Weight", towards the end of the section "Are you Yin?").

Then consult the Ch'ang Ming Health Diet Sheet (in Chapter 10 above) and the recommendations associated with it. In particular, remember:

1 no sugar whatsoever;
2 no tropical fruit (or drinks made from them), and only very occasionally local grown fruit;
3 reduce your salt intake;
4 don't boil your vegetables—sauté them;
5 reduce your fluid intake;
6 no cold food and no cold drinks;
7 cut out all milk products, including skimmed milk;
8 drink only herb teas, especially dandelion, fennel, nettle, sage, rosemary and China teas; and
9 eat eggs only scrambled or in omelettes.

The Chinese Cultural Arts Association will be pleased to hear from you if you care to drop a line saying how you have managed with your diet and how much surplus weight you have lost.

Chapter 13

Ladies—This is for You

As soon as she starts to menstruate, there is one question that every woman should ask herself: am I Yin or am I Yang? At that age she is not really old enough fully to appreciate what this means, and so it is up to her parents to let her know, as well as explain to her the workings of her body. If your own parents did not understand the Yin and Yang principles, you can at least ensure that any daughter of yours is properly informed.

Are you Yin?

Menstruation is a thing a woman tolerates because it will happen to her whether she likes it or not, and generally it is something she wishes that she had never been born to. What she goes through is, though, entirely in her own hands, for, if she suffers terrible pains, cramps, bad discharge, tumours, cysts, irregular periods and even frigidity, it is usually only because she does not realise that she can easily alter things for the better.

First of all, she should check a few facts concerning herself. She will probably find that she menstruates either at the time of the new moon (Yang) or between the new moon and the full moon (Yin). She may also find that she has irregular and sometimes long periods, generally at intervals of thirty to thirty-five days, that leave her very weak and listless. At times she will get excessive flow, coupled with abdominal pains and menstruation cramps, which are caused by bad eating habits, which lead to poor circulation (a sign of which is cold feet), which leads to congestion in the veins. At times there may also be a strong odour, which she may try to hide by the use of more powder, perfume and body sprays. She may even find that she becomes frigid after a while, as a result of internal contraction. To make things easier for herself at this awkward time, she should not wash her head and she should not have any cold baths or showers. A quick hot bath is all she needs, and it will do wonders to tone up the system generally.

Discharge. If the vaginal discharge is quite heavy at times, this is entirely owing to excess fat deposits inside the vagina, uterus, fallopian tubes, and even in and around the ovary. The colour of the discharge may vary and be either white, yellow or green; this is an important indicator of the internal health and should be watched most carefully.

A white discharge is a sign of too much fat. This is generally quite harmless, but if the excess persists over a long period a soft cyst may develop. This normally points to too much meat, sugar, tropical fruit, and dairy produce. The birth pill, if taken, will make the cyst more prominent and speed up its growth, and may cause many more such cysts to appear.

A yellow discharge is a worse sign, for it shows that there is an excess of fat inside the sexual organs and that the fat is turning rancid, as toxins and acids are produced. This is a clear warning that cysts could form if nothing is done to prevent it, and that the vagina is contracting sharply. This contraction is likely to be accompanied by spasms or stomach cramps. A sign of a very severe contraction is that after intercourse the man may find it difficult to withdraw. Such contraction can cause such a strain on the muscular system that the tissues lose their elasticity and their strength to hold and support, and internally everything becomes very loose, perhaps heading to the collapse of the uterus.

A colour of which to be especially wary about, is green. If the discharge is this colour for a long period of time, there is no doubt whatsoever that cancer could develop, unless something is done about it quickly.

All three colours indicate stages of Yin. If you want to do something about the trouble before it turns into something more serious, then start on a Ch'ang Ming diet straight away, and use sesame-seed salt or soya sauce with your meals.

Compresses (especially the ginger compress) are very useful for stimulating the circulation, breaking up fat deposits and dispersing cysts. For these purposes they should be used daily. Also very helpful are regular hip baths; and it is wise to douche regularly.

Pregnancy. All mothers will know of the various little changes that go on in their lives when they become pregnant. Menstruation ceases, sometimes there is irritability and restlessness, the taste-buds change and there is a yearning for foods out of season. The breasts start to become bigger and the nipples are tender to the touch. Morning sickness at this time is a Yin characteristic.

Bleeding during pregnancy is an indication that the blood capillaries in the uterus and the womb have become swollen by too much liquid and fruit and have exploded; it is a sure sign that the tissues are weak throughout your entire body, for if they were truly healthy they would be able to expand and contract without breaking. Weakness of the tissues is Yin and will be passed on to the baby in the womb. Miscarriages and premature births are suffered by very Yin mothers. The tendencies and feelings that the mother experiences during her pregnancy will be passed on to the child, whether they be laziness, irritability and aggressiveness or peace, tranquillity and happiness. It is in the mother's own hands to ensure for herself a happy and healthy child, by ensuring that she is happy and healthy too.

Further Yin signs are long, agonising labour pains, caused by muscular contraction, and a long delivery time (four to six hours) and painful birth. Breech births (where the feet come out first) and Caesarean operations (cutting through the walls of the abdomen to aid the delivery) are very, very Yin.

What an enormous responsibility parents have for the future health of their unborn children! This applies not only to the mother but also to the father, for if he drinks alcohol or takes drugs, this can affect the sperm and can radically affect the child during ovulation. If he loses his temper and upsets the mother while she is carrying, this too can have a detrimental effect on the unborn child.

Are you Yang?

If you menstruate at the time of the full moon then you are Yang and your periods will follow a regular cycle of twenty-eight days. You will also find that your flow will last only about three days, in which case the body will spend the next two days repairing itself. The loss of blood, and thus of energy, will be much smaller than with Yin menstruation. The flow should be quite light and thin, and there should be no clots and, thus, no pain. If however, the blood is very thick or it is only twenty-four days between menstruations, then you are far too Yang, so cut down a little on the amount of Yang foods that you are consuming, and also reduce slightly your intake of food. There should be no colour at all in your discharge, which should look like a thin transparent film of mucus, and there should be no smell or odour either.

Pregnancy. It takes about two and a half years to grow one layer of skin tissue, so if you want your blood and skin to be really healthy and to be able to have a baby completely naturally, with all the goodness within it that only nature can give, then start preparing for pregnancy at least three years in advance.

When you know that you are pregnant, make sure that your diet is absolutely in accordance with the guidelines of Ch'ang Ming, and don't break one single rule during the time that you are carrying. Also ensure that you have a quiet, restful, tranquil and happy time during the period that your baby is inside your womb, for love breeds love, and your baby will grow according to your own shadow.

You will find that you will have a very easy time during your pregnancy—no morning sickness, no unnecessary yearnings, no bleeding and hardly any inconvenience—and for most of the time you will feel so good that until the last few months you will scarcely notice that you are carrying. You will find that you carry your baby for the full nine months and part of the tenth month; so your baby will get the maximum benefit that you can pass on to it.

Ideally there should be no sexual intercourse at all during the time that the baby is being carried, but if there is mutual consent then it may occasionally be possible between the fifth and seventh months. The man, however, should be very careful and very gentle, and should not lie on top.

For the average Westerner the labour period lasts between eleven and sixteen hours, but for those on Ch'ang Ming it is eight to ten hours at the most, and when the time comes for delivery it is found to be painless and free of difficulties and lasting less than two hours (for those not on a Ch'ang Ming diet it usually lasts four hours or more). The head will be ready to come out first when the right time comes. The baby born of Ch'ang Ming parents will generally weigh about six pounds, which is complete goodness in a small package; the baby born to Yin parents, by contrast, will weigh rather more, the excess being made up of surplus fluids and toxins. Because of the extra weight of the Yin baby, the Yin mother (whose natural tendency is towards contraction) will find giving birth particularly difficult.

Warning. All prospective mothers should bear in mind the terrible lesson of the thalidomide tragedy; never use any drugs or medication, even if you have to have your baby in hospital. Make sure that you stress to the hospital authorities your wishes in this respect, and also make sure that only your own milk is given to your baby. This is very important, for in the first two or three days only colostrum comes out of your breasts, and this transparent, very Yang fluid will not only help your baby to become more Yang but also immunise your baby and enable it to fight off bacteria and many diseases. So give your baby a good start right from the very beginning, and remember that if you take any drugs they will be fed to your baby through your milk, so weakening, instead of strengthening, its health, and upsetting its ability to fight off infection.

Even though you are very strict with your diet and your baby is truly healthy, there is one disease that it will catch, and must catch, if it is really going to be fully Yang, and that is measles. This is one illness that is absolutely necessary for the child's expansion and physical growth, so the sooner it can contract it the better it is in helping the Yang influence to take over.

If your child should suffer any skin complaint or mumps, then it is Yin, for if it is truly healthy it will not catch these complaints at all.

Abdominal cramps are caused through over-consumption of Yin foods and fluids, which lead to congestion of the veins (this may also affect the legs, as a lot of women know already). Compresses will help relieve the condition and will also help to dissolve cysts. Use them whenever you can, and you will find that you receive great benefit from their use.

The most effective compress of all is the ginger compress, but if you have no ginger an onion compress is good, or failing that a cabbage compress, or failing that a salt-water compress. Since ginger is best, and penetrates deeply, it is worth buying some as soon as you can if you have none already.

Hip baths. (Tat'ui Hsitsao) have many excellent uses and can relieve many complaints, especially those to which women are prone. They are recommended as treatment for congestions, dysentry, poor circulation, irregular menstruation, menstrual cramps and pains, internal inflammations, leucorrhoea, and surplus fat around the mid-riff. They also stimulate the ovary and counterbalance the Yin contraction of the pituitary gland. Water is very Yin, and because of this a hip bath (in which the top half of the body stays out of the water) is not so weakening as a full immersion. Furthermore, you have a Yang heat influence working on a Yin illness.

To gain the maximum benefit from a hip bath, make sure that the water in the bath comes up no further than the navel, keep the water hot by adding a little extra hot water from time to time, wrap an old towel round your shoulders to help you to perspire more freely, and ensure that you sit in the bath for at least half an hour at a time. Don't catch cold afterwards, but keep yourself well wrapped up—better still, go straight to bed after you have dried yourself. If you take a hip bath every night for two weeks, you will be surprised how much your health benefits. The following are the best types of hip bath:

ginger hip bath (Chiang Tat'ui Hsitsao),
radish–salt hip bath (Luopo Hsien Tat'ui Hsitsao),
salt hip bath (Hsien Tat'ui Hsitsao),
eucalyptus hip bath (Anshu Tat'ui Hsitsao),
motherwort hip bath (Imu Ts'ao Tat'ui Hsitsao).

Teas. There are many very fine herb teas (Ts'ao Ch'a) suitable for treating the illnesses that Yin complaints cause in the Western woman, and it is certainly worth trying some. At first you may find that certain ones are not entirely to your taste, but give yourself time to get used to them, and if you like, add a little honey, soya sauce, cinnamon, clove or licorice as extra flavouring. The following are the teas most suitable for the complaints in question (which, if you keep to a strict Ch'ang Ming diet, will not trouble you anyway).

1 Sage (Tan Shen). Helps to promote regular menstruation, eases abdominal pain and invigorates the blood.
2 Hawthorn (Shan Cha). The roots and fruits are used to combat menstruation cramps, and to stop diarrhoea and dysentry.
3 Fennel (Hui Hsiang). Stimulates milk production.
4 Mugwort (Ai Yen). Effective in treating irregular menstruation. Disperses abdominal cramps and restores energy.
5 Dates (Ts'ao). Helps to combat fatigue and low energy levels.
6 Licorice (Kants'ao). Effective in treating irregular menstruation.
7 China Tea (Chungkuo Ch'a). Good for the circulation.
8 Cinnamon (Kuei Chih). Good for abdominal cramps.

Chapter 14

Grow Old Gracefully

How old is old? There are many in the West who at fifty already look as if they are preparing for the grave, when they have only reached the halfway stage of their true life. The Chinese believe that you are only at the *beginning* of old age when you are seventy years old, and that old age should be a time of great happiness, joy, spiritual understanding, and above all else, freedom.

At seventy you should reap the rewards of life, of having brought up the children and caring for them through thick and thin and then seeing them married and bearing children of their own. Through all this your love and understanding, and the help and guidance that you are able to give by virtue of your experience, can be enormous assistance to the whole family.

If you have obeyed the laws of the universe and have carefully kept to a Ch'ang Ming diet through your life then you will have no great problems to face when you reach your seventieth year. You will already have laid down the dynamic foundations for a long and prosperous old age.

You will have the stamina of the young, the healthy looks of the mature, the experience of the old, and, in addition to all this, the intuition, perception, internal tranquillity, positive and constant good health that only living close to nature over many, many years can bring. You will have attained the freedom of the universe at long last.

Those who are already fifty to sixty years of age are not too old to achieve full natural health and attain a degree of fulfilment that may previously have seemed far beyond their reach. Indeed, no one should consider himself too old to start on the road. Start on a Ch'ang Ming diet straight away, but be very strict with yourself, and take particular note of the following important points, which are especially for *YOU*:

1 Cut out all salt, and use soya sauce in its place.
2 Cut out all fat, and all foods that contain fat.
3 Never consume any tropical fruit or drinks made from it.

4 Reduce the amount of fluid that you drink daily.
5 Take extra care to chew your food thoroughly at every meal. Try to chew each mouthful of food until it turns to water.
6 Never consume any ice-cold food or drink.

At the end of two months you will be amazed at the progress in your health, and how much better you feel and look, and at the end of six months you will begin to look forward with great anticipation to the many happy years that lie ahead.

Instead of your family having to look after you, you will be the backbone of them all, and will be doing the most natural thing in the world: looking after *them*.

International Taoist Society

'The Chestnuts',
296 Bedford Road,
Rushden,
Northants.

You may be interested to know that this Society was formed on the foundations that were originally laid down by Professor Chan Kam Lee, who started the first Chinese Taoist Arts School in London in 1930.

Professor Lee died in the winter of 1953-4, when his boat sank, in a storm, off the coast of China, and it was then that his nephew Chee Soo was asked to take over the Presidency of all the Taoists Arts that were being taught. In 1958 Chee Soo set up the Coaching Classes with the object of training qualified teachers, county and National Coaches. Over the years these have been very successful and there are now classes and clubs operating in many parts of the world, besides those that exist in the British Isles.

Only the Taoist Arts of 'The Eight Strands of the Brocade' are taught within our Society and these comprise:

Ch'ang Ming	– Taoist Long Life Dietary Health Therapy
Ts'ao Yao	– Taoist Herbal Therapy
An Mo	– Taoist Massage
Tao Yin	– Taoist Respiration Therapy
Tien Chen	– Taoist Spot Pressing (Acupressure)
Ch'ili Nung	– Ch'i, Li, Vibration and Palm Healing
Chen Tuan	– Taoist Diagnosis Techniques

There are also two associations who are federated members of our Society:

The Chinese Cultural Arts Association who teach:

T'ai Chi Ch'uan	– The Supreme Ultimate
K'ai Men	– Taoist Yoga or the Taoist form of Chi Kung
I Fu Shou	– Sticky or Adhering Hands

Li Kung	– Taoist development of Li energy
Mo Kun	– Taoist Wand for external energy control
Mo Hsiang	– Taoist Meditation

also T'ai Chi Sword, T'ai Chi Sabre and T'ai Chi stick.

The International Wu Shu Association who teach:

Feng Shou	– 'Hand of the Wind' Kungfu, soft, gentle and fast, suitable for all ages
Chi Shu	– Taoist form of Aikido

and all the other forms of Taoist fighting arts including weapons.

Needless to say, all these associations strictly maintain the traditions that were laid down by Prof. Chan Kam Lee and his family.

Our President, Chee Soo, naturally, is also a Taoist, and his whole life is dedicated to serving and helping humanity whenever possible.

Anyone interested in any of these arts can attend any of the student coaching classes which are held regularly throughout the British Isles and in Europe. Details of these and of the classes and clubs that are available can be had from –

J. Harford (Mrs)
Courses Secretary

Index